Management of Clinical Depression and Anxiety

PSYCHO-ONCOLOGY CARE SERIES: COMPANION GUIDES FOR CLINICIANS

Published and Forthcoming Books in the Psycho-Oncology Care Series

Management of Clinical Depression and Anxiety

Psycho-Oncology in Palliative and End-of-Life Care

Sexual Health and Relationships

Cancer Survivorship and Health Promotion

Management of Clinical Depression and Anxiety

Edited By

Maggie Watson, PhD
Royal Marsden NHS Trust
Research Department of Clinical, Health and Educational Psychology
University College London
London, UK

David W. Kissane, MD
Department of Psychiatry
Monash University
Monash Medical Centre and Szalmuk Family Psycho-Oncology Unit
Cabrini Medical Centre
Melbourne, Australia

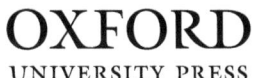

OXFORD
UNIVERSITY PRESS

OXFORD
UNIVERSITY PRESS

Oxford University Press is a department of the University of Oxford. It furthers the University's objective of excellence in research, scholarship, and education by publishing worldwide. Oxford is a registered trade mark of Oxford University Press in the UK and certain other countries.

Published in the United States of America by Oxford University Press
198 Madison Avenue, New York, NY 10016, United States of America.

© Oxford University Press 2017

All rights reserved. No part of this publication may be reproduced, stored in a retrieval system, or transmitted, in any form or by any means, without the prior permission in writing of Oxford University Press, or as expressly permitted by law, by license, or under terms agreed with the appropriate reproduction rights organization. Inquiries concerning reproduction outside the scope of the above should be sent to the Rights Department, Oxford University Press, at the address above.

You must not circulate this work in any other form
and you must impose this same condition on any acquirer.

Library of Congress Cataloging-in-Publication Data
Names: Watson, M., editor. | Kissane, David W. (David William), editor.
Title: Management of clinical depression and anxiety / edited by
Maggie Watson, David W. Kissane.
Description: New York, NY : Oxford University Press, [2017] |
Includes bibliographical references and index.
Identifiers: LCCN 2016030666 | ISBN 9780190491857 (pbk.)
Subjects: | MESH: Depressive Disorder—therapy | Anxiety Disorders—therapy
Classification: LCC RC537 | NLM WM 171.5 | DDC 616.85/27—dc23
LC record available at https://lccn.loc.gov/2016030666

This material is not intended to be, and should not be considered, a substitute for medical or other professional advice. Treatment for the conditions described in this material is highly dependent on the individual circumstances. And, while this material is designed to offer accurate information with respect to the subject matter covered and to be current as of the time it was written, research and knowledge about medical and health issues is constantly evolving and dose schedules for medications are being revised continually, with new side effects recognized and accounted for regularly. Readers must therefore always check the product information and clinical procedures with the most up-to-date published product information and data sheets provided by the manufacturers and the most recent codes of conduct and safety regulation. The publisher and the authors make no representations or warranties to readers, express or implied, as to the accuracy or completeness of this material. Without limiting the foregoing, the publisher and the authors make no representations or warranties as to the accuracy or efficacy of the drug dosages mentioned in the material. The authors and the publisher do not accept, and expressly disclaim, any responsibility for any liability, loss or risk that may be claimed or incurred as a consequence of the use and/or application of any of the contents of this material.

All case studies have been anonymized to protect patient identity.

Preface

Psycho-oncology is a subspecialty of oncology that focuses on psychosocial problems experienced by cancer patients and their families and carers; it provides evidence-based approaches to management of these specific problems.

The companion guides in the *Psycho-Oncology Care Series* are intended to make clinical management information accessible to either oncology clinical staff, who may not have had specialized mental health training, or those professionals still in training as mental health specialists seeking to increase their psycho-oncology skills.

Mental health problems in cancer patients can be both preexisting and arise within the context of the cancer's diagnosis and treatment. This companion guide covers clinical depression and anxiety and provides information relating to diagnosis, treatment, and service issues presented in a brief condensed format, which can be used as a quick access source to support clinical decision-making.

The authors of this Companion Guide are experienced clinicians and researchers with many years of experience in the care of patients with cancer and families. We thank them for sharing this expertise. As editors, we also thank the staff of Oxford University Press for their support and the International Psycho-Oncology Society for its assistance with distribution.

The psychosocial care of cancer patients and their families is a basic human right. We hope that the readers of this book will find it helpful to advance the quality of this care delivery to thus enrich the lives of all patients with cancer and their families.

Maggie Watson, PhD
David W. Kissane, MD

Contents

Contributors *ix*

1. **Distress, Adjustment, and Anxiety Disorders** *1*
   Daniel McFarland and Jimmie C. Holland

2. **Depression in Cancer Care** *23*
   Daisuke Fujisawa and Yosuke Uchitomi

3. **Diagnosis and Treatment of Demoralization** *42*
   David W. Kissane

4. **Recognizing and Managing Suicide Risk** *61*
   Maggie Watson and Luigi Grassi

5. **Psychopharmacologic Management of Anxiety and Depression** *78*
   Madeline Li, Joshua Rosenblat, and Gary Rodin

   Appendix 1: NCCN Distress Thermometer and Problem List *109*
   Appendix 2: Demoralization Scale-II *111*
   Appendix 3: Brief Screening Tools *112*
   Appendix 4: Tools for the Assessment of Suicide Risk *113*
   Appendix 5: Answers to Chapter Quizzes *114*

   Index *117*

Contributors

Daisuke Fujisawa, MD, PhD
Department of Neuropsychiatry and Palliative Care Center
Keio University School of Medicine
Tokyo, Japan

Luigi Grassi, MD
Institute of Psychiatry
Department of Biomedical and Specialty Surgical Sciences
University of Ferrara
Hospital Psychiatry Unit
S. Anna University Hospital and Health Authorities
Ferrara, Italy

Jimmie C. Holland, MD
Department of Psychiatry and Behavioral Sciences
Memorial Sloan-Kettering Cancer Center
New York, NY

David W. Kissane, MD
Department of Psychiatry
Monash University
Monash Medical Centre and Szalmuk Family Psycho-Oncology Unit
Cabrini Medical Centre
Melbourne, Australia

Madeline Li, MD, PhD
Department of Supportive Care
University Health Network—Princess Margaret Cancer Centre
Toronto, Canada

Daniel McFarland, DO
Division of Regional Network Services
Department of Medicine
Memorial Sloan-Kettering Cancer Center
West Harrison, NY

Gary Rodin, MD
Department of Supportive Care
University Health Network—Princess Margaret Cancer Centre
Toronto, Canada

Joshua Rosenblat, MD
Department of Psychiatry
University Health Network—Princess Margaret Cancer Centre
Toronto, Canada

Yosuke Uchitomi, MD, PhD
Innovation Center for Supportive, Palliative and Psychosocial Care
Department of Psycho-Oncology
National Cancer Center Hospital
Tokyo, Japan

Maggie Watson, PhD
Royal Marsden NHS Trust
Research Department of Clinical, Health and Educational Psychology
University College London
London, UK

Management of Clinical Depression and Anxiety

Chapter 1

Distress, Adjustment, and Anxiety Disorders

Daniel McFarland and Jimmie C. Holland

Learning Objectives

After reading this chapter, the clinician will be able to
1. Provide background that will help him or her assimilate and contextualize distress, adjustment disorders, and formal anxiety disorders in patients with cancer.
2. Describe the presenting problems. This includes grasping the diagnostic dilemmas and therapeutic applicability between these clinical disorders to provide quality supportive care for patients with cancer and their families.
3. Outline key investigations for making a diagnosis. The clinician should be able to describe the most useful investigations for distinguishing between differential diagnoses.
4. Describe clinical management options. The clinician should be able to appreciate the management decisions and available clinical options.
5. Clarify professional issues in managing distress and anxiety disorders in the cancer setting.

Background Evidence

Cancer frequently causes emotional turmoil for patients and families. Its psychological symptoms may be just as insidious or extreme as its physical symptoms, but historically they have largely gone unrecognized. Increasingly recognized is the prevalence of distress and/or psychiatric disorders in approximately 30% to 60% of patients newly diagnosed with various types of cancer.[1-3] Psychological disturbances may present at any time but with increased frequency at certain points in the cancer trajectory: at diagnosis, with cancer recurrence or progression, and during advanced cancer states or survivorship.[4] Clinician barriers to the identification of distress include a perceived lack of time, inadequate training or interview skills, a low index of suspicion, and low awareness of mental health complications.[1]

Distress

Distress was chosen as a word to use with patients because it did not cause embarrassment. It can serve as an umbrella term for the range of emotional problems that arise during a patient's illness in response to physical symptoms, sadness, worry, or concerns for family or one's own existence as well as severe symptoms of depression and anxiety. The National Comprehensive Cancer Network (NCCN) noted in 1996 that distress has multiple causes related to physical, social, psychological (e.g., concern for family), and existential or spiritual concerns. Although a clinical assessment is always necessary for a complete evaluation of distress, several validated scales are used to identify those patients who would benefit from further psychological care. The most commonly used measure is the NCCN Distress Thermometer and Problem List (DT&PL), similar to the zero to 10 Likert scale that has been successfully implemented for pain management (see Appendix 1 on p. 109). In 2008, the Institute of Medicine's report *Cancer Care for the Whole Patient: Meeting Psychosocial Health Needs* noted there was a sufficient evidence base for both psychosocial and psychopharmacologic interventions to necessitate a policy statement that quality cancer care must integrate psychosocial treatments into routine cancer treatment.[5] In 2010, the International Psycho-Oncology Society (IPOS) and the International Union Against Cancer endorsed its use as the sixth vital sign, after pain.

Adjustment Disorders

Here symptoms occur in reaction to the stressor of cancer and are considered disproportionate or excessive. The development of impairment in interpersonal, social, or occupational areas of functioning is central to the diagnosis. This distinction requires clinical judgment, as receiving a cancer diagnosis is stressful under most circumstances and adjustment disorders are the least studied entities in the American Psychiatric Association's *Diagnostic and Statistical Manual of Mental Disorders* (DSM). However, they are by far the most commonly diagnosed psychiatric disorders in patients with cancer.[1] Its previous stand-alone categorization in the fourth edition of the DSM did not encourage research in this area. The fifth edition of the DSM has placed adjustment disorders under the "Trauma and Stressor-Related Disorders" category, which makes the relationship to the stressor of cancer clearer and may potentiate research to understand and delineate it better. The lack of specificity, aside from a reaction to a stressor, should cause the clinician to expand the differential diagnosis and consider alternate diagnoses (e.g., demoralization).

Anxiety Disorders

Although anxiety is pervasive in patients with cancer, the prevalence rates of specific anxiety disorders are less well defined.[6] The majority of anxiety experienced in the setting of cancer is situational and not debilitating. It may be classified as an adjustment disorder with anxious features or as an anxiety disorder due to a general medical condition.[7] In addition, various medical situations in the cancer trajectory may exacerbate anxiety, or it may be comorbid with depression or cancer (e.g., uncontrolled pain, medication side effect, dyspnea, nausea).[8,9] Anxiety is a normal response to cancer and can even be helpful for some people who take steps to reduce the anxiety (e.g., information-seeking, reaching out for social support). More significant anxiety disorders are typically present before the cancer diagnosis and may be identified as a generalized anxiety disorder, panic disorder, phobia, or post-traumatic stress disorder (PTSD).[10]

A high-quality oncology practice requires the recognition and treatment of comorbid distress and anxiety in accordance with clinical practice guidelines. The oncology team on the "front line" is central to delivering quality psychosocial cancer care. This high-quality, evidence-based management strategy essentially requires a truly "caring" approach that fosters a trusting therapeutic relationship, as trust is influential in determining clinical outcomes. This chapter outlines the management of these symptoms in accordance with these principles.

Presenting Problems

Fear

Fear is a reaction to a known threat. It may be provoked by the inevitability of death, uncertainty, worry about proposed treatments, or negative reactions from treating physicians, nurses, and other staff members, for example.

Anxiety

Anxiety is a reaction to both real and imagined threats. It may be provoked by the uncertainty of the cancer prognosis or even the diagnosis itself (5% to 10% of cancers are unknown primary), the impact of the illness on one's identity and livelihood, the effects on one's body, or anxiety about interacting with strangers or being alone in the hospital. At the same time, anxiety in the cancer setting may not be directly related to cancer. For example, in the face of a cancer diagnosis or recurrence, a primary anxiety or mood disorder may be exacerbated or one may worry about interpersonal relationships. The diagnosis may exacerbate a patient's social situation, which then impairs psychic equilibrium (e.g., financial instability, spousal and/or family interactions). Patients with cognitive impairment or dementia frequently experience anxiety with changes in daily routines.

Coping

Patients may convey a sense of poor coping. Understanding "normal," adaptive reactions to the cancer stressor helps the clinician to determine what might be a pathological response (see Box 1.1). A sense of poor coping may vary over the course of the illness as well (e.g., acute anxiety at diagnosis, chronic anxiety related to the fear of recurrence or hereditary genetic testing) or may be comorbidly present with depression or a medical condition (e.g., uncontrolled pain, medication side effect, dyspnea, nausea) and remit with medical attention. At the same time, patients may develop a de novo anxiety disorder during the cancer trajectory.

> **Box 1.1 Issues Complicating the Presentation of Distress and Anxiety in the Cancer Setting**
>
> - Clinicians do not recognize impaired functioning and pathological symptoms
> - Patients underreport their symptoms
> - Differences in cancer center psychosocial resource allotment
> - Diagnostic confusion with medical conditions

Stigma and Masked Distress

Patients may conceal or minimize symptoms that they feel are less important than dealing with the cancer. Also, they may fear that their oncologist may not treat them the same as other patients, fearing the stigma associated with a label of poor coping.

Physical Symptoms

Tremor, palpitations, sweating, breathlessness, and hyperventilation can all be markers of anxiety. Patients with cancer can have numerous physical ailments that tend to change over time and complicate comorbid psychological symptoms or psychiatric diagnoses. Disorientation, confusion, and cognitive impairment may represent delirium. A patient with an intracranial mass (e.g., common in lung and breast cancers or a primary mass) or thyroid dysfunction (e.g., from a pituitary mass or endocrine tumor) may present with apathy or irritability and appear to be depressed or, conversely, could exhibit hyperactivity, disinhibition, or mania-like states. The underlying biological effects of anticancer treatments may also confound the psychological presentation.

Distress

This is defined by the NCCN as "an unpleasant experience of an emotional, psychological, social, or spiritual nature that interferes with the ability to cope with cancer treatment. It extends along a continuum, from common normal feelings of vulnerability, sadness, and fears, to problems that are disabling, such as true depression, anxiety, panic, and feeling isolated or in a spiritual crisis." It is identified by the patient and may or may not coincide with functional impairment. Patients experience distress and interpret its meaning in a variety of ways. It may be a healthy reaction to a stressor, or it may lead to functional impairment and can be a harbinger for future psychiatric complications during cancer treatments or into survivorship.

Assessment of Distress as the Presenting Problem

A patient's distress should always be assessed clinically, as it may or may not be associated with decreased function, which is an indication for a more significant intervention. The reason for distress is often discovered through use of an instrument (e.g., the problem list component of the DT&PL; see Appendix 1 on p. 109) in conjunction with a clinical interview.

🔍 **Key Questions:**
- How have you been dealing with the stress of the diagnosis?
- How has it affected your life?
- How would those who are close to you say you are doing?
- Is there anything that you are no longer able to do because of its impact on your life?
- Do you feel safe and in control?

Problem List

Screening with a valid instrument is encouraged but should always be followed up with a clinical assessment (see Box 1.2). Although the NCCN recommends the DT&PL, there is not one accepted gold standard for distress screening. Researchers have advocated for a two-step screening with the DT&PL and another short screening measure, such as the Hospital Anxiety and Depression Scale (HADS).

Vulnerability Factors

The NCCN distress guidelines define time points when assessments for distress, adjustment disorders, and anxiety should be made. Certain time points in the cancer trajectory may exacerbate anxiety (e.g., at initial diagnosis, in anticipation of check-ups, during diagnostic studies that might detect recurrence, with advancing disease, with news of a poor prognosis, or at the end of active treatment, when surveillance intervals are increased). Special attention should be placed on distress screening at the cancer diagnosis, at recurrence, or during any vulnerable period (see Box 1.3); every six months; and into the survivorship period. The best method of triaging is one of the crucial issues with regard to initiating a comprehensive appraisal of patients with cancer.

Box 1.2 Patients at Increased Risk for Distress as Identified by the NCCN

- History of psychiatric disorder/substance abuse
- History of depression/suicide attempt
- Cognitive impairment
- Severe comorbid illnesses
- Uncontrolled cancer-related symptoms
- Spiritual/religious concerns
- Social issues (e.g., family/caregiver conflicts, inadequate social support, living alone, financial problems, limited access to medical care, young or dependent children, younger age, female, history of abuse [physical, sexual], other stressors)

Adapted with permission from the NCCN.

Box 1.3 NCCN Designated Periods of Increased Vulnerability

- Finding a suspicious symptom
- During a diagnostic workup
- At diagnosis
- Awaiting treatment, changing treatment modalities, or at the end of treatment
- Significant treatment-related complication(s) or treatment failure
- Discharge from the hospital following treatment
- Transition to survivorship
- Recurrence/progression
- Advanced cancer conditions, and at end of life.

Adapted with permission from the NCCN.

Comprehensive Psychiatric Workup

It is essential to thoroughly review a patient's psychosocial issues and also to ensure that a complete medical workup has been performed. A previous psychiatric history may antedate and help to elucidate the manifestation of ongoing events, for example. Once distress has been identified and established with the patient, a comprehensive interview process should begin. Some key questions to begin the interview process are listed in Box 1.4.

Once distress-related issues are identified, a comprehensive interview should follow. Its integral components consist of a review of the present social support system (e.g., key relationships or their absence), social history (family, friends, occupation, hobbies, habits/addictions), development history (e.g., education, life-course milestones), and present functional impairment in daily or otherwise important activities. Clinical assessments should be made in a confidential manner that enhances or builds trust. They should

Box 1.4 Comprehensive Psychiatric Workup—Key Questions to Ask Distressed Patients

- Help me to better understand your distress. What is it that worries you the most?
- Are there other sources of anxiety?
- What aspect of your illness is most frightening?
- Are there physical symptoms that make it hard to cope?
- Do you have a past history of anxiety or chronic worry?
- How has your sleep been? What happens when you try to sleep?
- Do you have any symptoms of panic? tension? restlessness? tremor? any other symptoms of concern?
- Does all that you've been describing spoil your quality of life? interfere with your activities and how you function?

> **Box 1.5 Distress Screening Overview**
> - Distress screening and psychological assessment at NCCN-designated time points and whenever symptoms arise
> - Comprehensive clinical interview (e.g., reviewing social and development history and present functional impairment)
> - Assess for safety
> - Treatment interventions (psychological/pharmacologic)
> - Treatment intervention follow-up/assess for titration
> - Assess treatment effects at follow-up subsequent visits

be reassuring, comprehensive, and not hurried. The conversation should be allowed to flow in the direction of concern for the patient. The clinician should work to minimize stigma by paying attention to word choice and opting for words such as *distress, concerns, worries, uncertainties,* or *stressors* and avoid words such as *psychiatric, psychological, mental disorder, maladjustment,* or *mental illness*. An overview of distress screening is provided in Box 1.5.

Clinical Management

Nonspecific Distress

The management of distress should be problem-focused and directed toward ameliorating the cause of distress, if possible, in addition to symptom-directed management. Guidance from the primary medical team to fully assess the effects of an intervening medical or medication-related cause for the patient's symptoms is vitally important. In addition, a formal psychiatric diagnosis should be ruled out, depending on the safety assessment and severity of symptoms. The problem list that accompanies the DT&PL can be helpful in identifying the cause of distress along with a problem-focused clinical interview. (See the "Assessment of Distress as the Presenting Problem" section for details of the clinical interview assessment.) Referrals should be made to the appropriate clinician in order to obtain a comprehensive assessment. For instance, a social worker may best address financial issues and a chaplain may best address spiritual issues.

In general, acknowledging patient distress is the beginning of a therapeutic intervention. Many patients benefit simply from reviewing and clarifying information about their diagnosis, treatment options, and side effects. Frequently, patients receive information from various professional and lay sources that may run counter to their understanding.

Some key considerations for troubleshooting distress are
- Review how to interpret the information that is gathered in the medical system.
- Always assess for patient understanding and refer to appropriate sources (e.g., NCCN Treatment Summaries for Patients).

- Counsel patients on how to mobilize and avail themselves of resources. Ensuring continuity of care can also be highly therapeutic and help to establish rapport.
- Offer guidance on securing the following services (depending on need):
  - Counseling (e.g., support groups, family or individual counseling)
  - Symptom-directed interventions (e.g., relaxation techniques such as guided imagery, meditation, or creative art/music therapies)
  - Spiritual support
  - Exercise interventions
- Use collateral information and follow-up patient interviews to assess the need to escalate care.
- Re-evaluate after prescribed interventions.

Standards for distress management have been developed by the NCCN (see www.nccn.org/professionals/physician_gls/f_guidelines.asp). Distress should be recognized, monitored, documented, and treated promptly at all stages of disease and in all settings. The NCCN suggests that interdisciplinary committees review institutional standards for distress management. The training of professionals in distress screening is mandatory in order to ensure the proliferation of skill sets.

Case Study

Distress Management

Frank was diagnosed with prostate cancer two years ago after routine surveillance detected an elevated prostate-specific antigen (PSA). He opted for a surgical approach to treat his localized prostate cancer and underwent a radical prostatectomy. He tolerated the surgery well without significant postoperative complications and was able to urinate without difficulty and achieve erections. His urologist has been following his PSA and has noted a significant doubling time in less than six months. Imaging reveals no evidence of active prostate cancer, but it is recommended that Frank undergo local radiation to the operative site. He reports a distress level of 10 and identifies several emotional problems including nervousness, sadness, and fear and is concerned about the effects of radiation. He has many friends who have had terrible complications from radiation, including death. His clinician reviews his distress data and interviews Frank about his concerns. Frank feels devastated that the cancer has "come back," feels like he was not successful, and deeply fears the effects of radiation. The clinician decides to clarify that this "adjuvant" treatment will be done in order to prevent an actual cancer recurrence on imaging (i.e., Frank has a biochemical prostate cancer recurrence), and more patient-directed information packets are provided for Frank. It is decided that a staff member will follow up with Frank and that his distress will be assessed at the next visit. Frank tolerates the radiation well without complications and has subsequent distress levels between 1 and 3.

Adjustment Disorders

Adjustment disorders are the most commonly identified comorbid psychiatric diagnoses in the setting of cancer. They indicate poor coping.

Diagnostic criteria

Adjustment disorders are diagnosed when there are

- Symptoms (e.g., anxiety, excessive worry, sadness, hopelessness, loss of appetite) deemed to be in excess of what would be expected from the stressor.
- Social or occupational loss of function related to the stressor of cancer. The symptoms must cause significant impairment in social or occupational functioning within three months of the stressor.
- Symptoms that do not meet the criteria for another Axis I psychiatric disorder.

Key symptoms and signs

Situational symptoms are usually insomnia, worry, muscle tension, restlessness, dyspnea, dyspepsia, palpitations, sweating, being jittery or light-headed (i.e., with anxious features) or irritable, mood swings, and transient spells of hopelessness or demoralization (i.e., with mixed or depressive features). Tearfulness that is experienced as an emotional release suggests an adjustment disorder; crying with major depression is more likely to feel emotionally draining and not relieving for the patient. Transient fixation on cancer-related phenomena (i.e., tumor markers, "markeritis") might be indicative of an adjustment disorder.

Clinical perspective

Adjustment disorders can be either acute, if the disturbance lasts for less than six months, or chronic, if the disturbance lasts for six months or longer in the face of an ongoing stressor. The signs and symptoms of adjustment disorders are variable and can be masked by what either the patient or the clinician may consider a normal reaction to a cancer diagnosis, cancer recurrence, or living with cancer. Functionality in occupation or relationships is usually impaired in some way, and this may or may not be acknowledged by the patient. Collateral information from friends or family is frequently helpful, but the patient should identify cancer or treatment as the stressor.

Differential diagnosis

There is no an ideal questionnaire for diagnosing adjustment disorders in cancer patients. Measures such as the HADS, a brief, 14-item self-report scale, can be used to assess and monitor distressed patients with advanced disease or other medical conditions. A combined score in excess of 10 suggests an adjustment disorder; 20 or higher suggests major depression.

Treatment

Psychotherapy. This should be considered for all adjustment disorders; it should focus on restoring the patient's functional ability and address coping with the stressor if possible (see Figure 1.1). In the cancer setting, clarifying a realistic understanding of the seriousness of the diagnosis and prognosis is key. Therapy may then focus on adapting, accepting, adjusting the interpretation, and finding meaning in the experience. Appropriate therapies should be directed toward the amelioration of symptoms and supporting coping resources. This may be best done by problem-solving or ameliorating

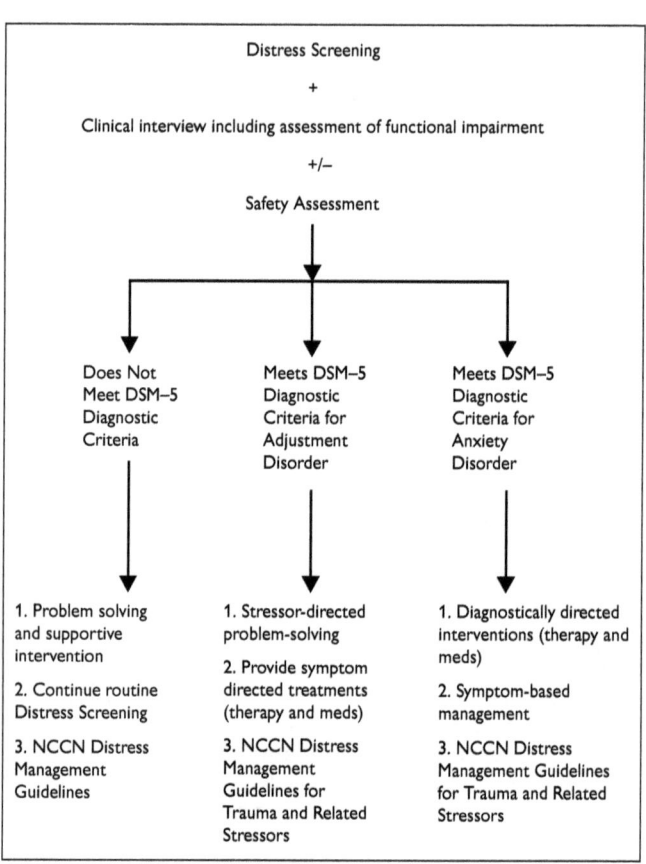

Figure 1.1. Overall management algorithm for distress and anxiety in cancer care. Adapted with permission from the NCCN guidelines.

symptoms with supportive counseling and/or psychopharmacology. The management should be patient-directed and in accordance with his or her preferences for treatment but with explicit professional guidance. Also, assessments for safety and excluding other Axis I psychiatric disorders are imperative (see Box 1.6).

Educating patients, controlling physical symptoms, and maintaining effective communication are essential therapeutic tools that restore patients' innate coping abilities. In addition to discussing concerns, patients may benefit from participating in a support group or a supportive-expressive psychotherapy group that is problem-focused on current life problems with other patients. Cognitive behavioral therapy (CBT) may be effective for assessing overly negative or irrational interpretations and instituting symptom-directed behavioral interventions for insomnia and fatigue, for example. Psychological interventions are effective, and their implementation can even be taught to

> **Box 1.6 Types of Manual-Based Therapies Recommended in the IPOS *Handbook of Psychotherapy in Cancer Care***
>
> - CBT
> - Supportive-expressive therapy
> - Meaning-centered therapy
> - Psycho-educational interventions
> - Family-focused grief therapy
> - Guided writing
> - Narrative therapy
> - Mindfulness-based therapy
> - Reconstructing meaning and cognitive-analytic therapy
> - Motivational interviewing

nonmental health professionals in certain cases. This may be effective in certain cases since rather consistent evidence suggests that cancer patients prefer more support and communication directly from oncology clinical staff. For more information, see www.nccn.org/professionals/physician_gls/f_guidelines.asp.

Psychotropic medication. Consider this for moderate/severe adjustment disorders. Treat the patient symptomatically with a hypnotic to promote sleep or an anxiolytic to reduce worry. If there is no response to the medication, dosages should be titrated. (See chapter 5 for a complete discussion of medications. Here we only cover key principles.) If there is no subsequent response, another disorder with or without a personality disorder should be considered. After a response is achieved, patients should be followed, and there should be communication with the patient's family and primary oncology team. Treatment for any mood disorder should always consider an underlying medical etiology of the mood disturbance and be directed toward ameliorating the specific symptoms that are the most distressing (e.g., anhedonia, fatigue, insomnia, anorexia, suicidal thoughts) (see Box 1.7).

Adjustment disorders may be addressed with psychopharmacological treatment in order to target key symptoms such as in the amelioration of anxiety or insomnia. Anxiolytics provide relief from anxiety within one to

> **Box 1.7 Medical Causes of Mood Disturbance**
>
> - Sickness syndrome with advanced cancer states
> - Intracranial malignancy involvement
> - Electrolyte disturbances (e.g., elevated calcium)
> - Delirious states (e.g., from infection, treatment-related, postsurgical)
> - Medications (e.g., corticosteroids, interferon alpha, akathisia from neuroleptics)

several days, while antidepressants typically take from two to six weeks for therapeutic benefits in reducing panic or anxiety. Psychotropic prescriptions should be individualized to the patient and based on therapeutic tolerability. Classes of psychiatric medications used in adjustment disorders include the anxiolytics (e.g., benzodiazepines), hypnotics (e.g., zolpidem), antidepressants (selective serotonin reuptake inhibitors [SSRIs], serotonin–norepinephrine reuptake inhibitors [SNRIs], "atypical antidepressants," tricyclic antidepressants), and very rarely monoamine oxidase inhibitors and antipsychotic medications (e.g., olanzapine). The psychopharmacologic treatment of adjustment disorders specifically includes the short-term use of anxiolytics, hypnotics, and/or antidepressants.

Anxiolytics and their dose titration should be chosen based on the patient's level of anxiety and functional impairment, medical and/or substance use/abuse history, along with previous anxiolytic use. Benzodiazepines are the most commonly used anxiolytic. Starting doses should always be the lowest effective dose and should be titrated according to symptoms and tolerability (e.g., sedation, memory impairment). Caution should be exercised in patients with a substance abuse history or in the setting of dementia or cognitive impairment. Drug metabolism should be carefully considered in patients with liver or renal impairment. In general, short-acting benzodiazepines are safest to use in patients with liver impairment, while lorazepam is the safest to use in patients with renal failure. Alprazolam should be prescribed cautiously given its relative short half-life and potential to precipitate anxiety when effects wear off. Patients should be warned of the addictive potential and be weaned off these medications as soon as possible.

Antidepressant medications are effective in patients with panic disorder, and the choice of antidepressant should be guided by the side-effect profile (e.g., weight gain, anorexia, anxiogenic, sedative), the likelihood of serious adverse events, the potential for drug interactions with anticancer or other treatments, and the lethality of the medication in the case of a suicide attempt. For example, weight gain may be of particular concern for certain patient populations (e.g., breast cancer), where weight gain could adversely affect prognosis, versus a benefit in other scenarios (e.g., advanced cancer cachexia). The prescriber should also be concerned with interactions with other medications that are commonly used in the cancer setting. For example, the prescriber should be aware of the potential for the serotonin syndrome (e.g., interactions with hydrocodone, tramadol, metoclopramide, fentanyl, ondansetron, triptans), a bleeding diathesis with anticoagulation (e.g., SSRI antiplatelet effects), and metabolism of anticancer drugs (e.g., decreased levels of the tamoxifen metabolite, endoxifen, with 2D6 metabolizers).

Antidepressants should be evaluated for side effects and effectiveness over a course of two to six weeks. Titrations should be made based on the drug's tolerability and potential for therapeutic benefit. Drugs should be titrated at several-week intervals to reach an effect that is deemed beneficial by the patient. At the very least, a drug should be titrated to the recommended dose (e.g., escitalopram 20 mg daily). Also, patients should be started at the lowest doses and even half the recommended starting dose when they express particular concern about side effects. It is beneficial for patients to start at subtherapeutic antidepressant doses and gain confidence with the drug before titrating upward, especially as outpatients. If they are starting an antidepressant for the first time, a side effect or negative experience may deter them from taking the medication again in the future.

Medication choices and psychotherapy types for adjustment disorders should be prescribed based on patient characteristics and his or her life situation. These are generally short-term treatments in the setting of adjustment disorders.

Case Study

Adjustment Disorder Management

Mrs. M was diagnosed with extensive small cell lung cancer six weeks ago. She thinks about her new diagnosis constantly and frequently does not get up from her bed. She has sought medical options/opinions from three oncologists and has yet to start treatment. She worries about not having enough time to be with her children and/or complete other life tasks that she has identified as unfilled. She is divorced and recently unemployed. She fears her cancer diagnosis. She has been unable to stay asleep and remains fatigued during the day for the last week. She frequently feels better after crying spells and gets some relief from her close friends who have vowed to stay by her side. A comprehensive assessment reveals an excessive reaction to her diagnosis that is impairing her functioning (i.e., reluctant to commit to treatment) and that does not meet criteria for other psychiatric disorders, and her presentation is most accurately summarized by adjustment disorder with mixed features. She is encouraged to utilize her support system, obtains further information about her treatment options, takes a hypnotic to start sleeping, and will start escitalopram. She is accompanied by a friend to start chemotherapy. Six months after the diagnosis, her coping is restored and her relationships are well preserved.

Anxiety Disorders

Intense fear, an inability to absorb information, and an inability to cooperate with medical requests may be presenting features of an anxiety disorder. Anxiety leads to poor quality of life, independent of its association with depression. Although 34% of patients may have clinical anxiety symptoms, the majority of anxiety disorders in the cancer setting are a reactivation of a previously diagnosed disorder. Anxiety disorders can detract from patient-centered care as the patient may sabotage his or her involvement in medical decision-making or have multiple exacerbations of medical symptoms that lead to excessive workup and possibly more invasive tests and disruptions in cancer care. Psychosocial assessment may benefit from multidisciplinary input, and communication should be sought with the primary oncology team and consultants. Palliative care specialists may be able to provide expertise in the management of underlying pain or other physical, spiritual issues. Other specialties may provide insightful management in their areas of expertise. Also, primary care providers may be able to provide a unique assessment of psychosocial adjustment that may predate the cancer diagnosis.

Symptoms and signs

In general, symptoms of anxiety typically consist of cognitive, emotional, physical, and behavioral components. Cognitively, patients may fixate their focus on threats (e.g., cancer and otherwise), worry excessively, catastrophize, and underestimate their ability to cope. Emotionally, they may feel nervous, panicky, or just plain scared. Physically, they may experience breathlessness, chest tightness, palpitations, and GI discomfort (diarrhea/nausea), diaphoresis, or muscle tension. Behaviorally, patients may act in a way that avoids the immediate threat they fear, seek reassurance, or become paralyzed with anxiety.

Each type of anxiety disorder may present with the somatic signs of autonomic hyper-reactivity (e.g., shortness of breath, sweating, lightheadedness, palpitations), motor tension (e.g., restlessness, muscle tension, and fatigue), and/or vigilance (e.g., irritability, exaggerated startle response, feeling "on edge"; see Table 1.1).

Diagnostic criteria

The types of anxiety disorders that manifest in the cancer setting and can impact care are phobias, panic disorder, generalized anxiety disorder, PTSD,

Table 1.1 Signs and Symptoms of Anxiety

Anxiety Symptom Cluster	Description
Psychological	• Worry, apprehension, fear, and sadness • Patient may be able to identify focus or source of these symptoms • Often nonspecific and "free-floating" • Crying spells, ruminations • Typical complaint (especially at night): inability to "turn off" one's thoughts
Physical	• Tachycardia and tachypnea • Tremor, diaphoresis, nausea, dry mouth, insomnia, and anorexia
May be intermittent: increasing over hours or days	• In response to a stressor (e.g., anticipation of pending diagnostic testing or procedures) with resolution if/when the stressor passes
May be persistent and pervasive through the day	• Typical of primary anxiety disorders • Comorbid depressive disorders • Reactions to chronic stressors (e.g., fear of cancer recurrence, family/financial problems) • Side effects of regularly prescribed medications
Panic attacks present with paroxysmal acute anxiety	• Severe palpitations, diaphoresis, and nausea. There is often a sense of great fear of a catastrophic event, described as a "feeling of impending doom" • Usually lasts for at least several minutes. The frequency is variable with multiple possible events in a single day

and anxiety disorders caused by other general medical conditions. Highlights of specific anxiety disorders are given in Table 1.2.

Clinical perspective

- **Phobias**—The cancer setting may exacerbate specific phobias or previously unknown phobic reactions, and these can even escalate to sheer panic. For example, patients are placed in enclosed spaces (e.g., for an MRI) and sometimes for long periods of time (e.g., during a bone marrow transplant). Aside from claustrophobia, patients may have needle phobias during routine blood draws, after specific anticancer treatments (e.g., surgery), after complications (e.g., an ICU stay), or during routine doctor's visits (e.g., "white coat syndrome").
- **Chronic worriers**—Patients with generalized anxiety disorders have usually been chronic worriers their entire lives and will readily admit this, if asked.
- **Conditioned responses**—In the past, anxiety appeared as a conditioned response to chemotherapy that is highly emetogenic when control of nausea and vomiting was poor. Patients would become anxious from the smell of the antiseptic or the sight of the chemo infusion site staff. These conditions of avoidance can develop into a cancer-related PTSD. Other medically related conditions can be exacerbated in the cancer setting (e.g., congestive heart failure, seizures, complex regional pain syndromes) or appear for the first time (e.g., pulmonary embolism, myocardial infarction, seizures) and cause anxiety symptoms.

Differential diagnosis

The medical context must always be considered in the differential diagnosis, and a basic laboratory workup will help to elucidate organ dysfunction (renal, liver, bone marrow), risk of infection, or encephalopathy. This should include the following.

- Electrolytes and urea testing. Electrolyte disturbances that are a result of cancer (e.g., syndrome of inappropriate antidiuretic hormone, parathyroid hormone related protein, paraneoplastic syndromes, hormone-secreting tumors) or its treatment (e.g., excessive intravenous fluids, chemotherapy, induced vomiting such as with cisplatin) may cause or exacerbate delirium states and seizures.
- Full blood exam (look for anemia and neutrophilia for infection).
- Liver function tests to test for effect of malignancy and alcohol use.
- Thyroid test panel and/or cortisol or adrenal suppression test when necessary to test for hormonal disturbances.
- MRI or CT imaging as appropriate to test for brain or spinal cord masses.
- An electrocardiogram (EKG) to find present or underlying cardiac pathology. Anxiety symptoms may be the result of a pulmonary embolus that could be suggested on an EKG and seen on a CT chest x-ray with a pulmonary embolus protocol.
- Screening for several classes of medications that can cause and exacerbate anxiety and should be considered in the differential diagnosis of anxiety. Sympathomimetics (e.g., albuterol inhaler), corticosteroids that are used routinely with chemotherapy, immunosuppressants (e.g., cyclosporine),

Table 1.2 Anxiety Disorders and Cancer-Specific Considerations

Disorder	DSM-5 Diagnostic Features	Cancer-Specific Considerations
Specific Phobia	• Marked fear or anxiety about specific objects or situations that is difficult to control (e.g., needles, closed spaces) • Anxiety is associated with several symptoms (e.g., restlessness, fatigue, difficulty concentrating, irritability, muscle tension, and sleep problems)	• Worries may include perseveration on symptoms, disease course, scans, treatment outcomes, and loss of functioning • Difficulty concentrating may interfere with clinical communication and treatment decision-making
Generalized Anxiety Disorder	• At least six months of excessive worry about a number of events or activities, which is difficult to control • Anxiety is associated with several symptoms (e.g., restlessness, fatigue, difficulty concentrating, irritability, muscle tension, and sleep problems)	• Worries may include perseveration on symptoms, disease course, scans, treatment outcomes, side effects, role transitions, and loss of functioning • Difficulty concentrating may interfere with clinical communication and treatment decision-making
Panic Disorder	• Recurrent unexpected panic attacks that develop abruptly • Panic attack followed by at least one month of (a) persistent worry of having further panic attacks and/or (b) maladaptive change in behavior due to panic (e.g., avoidance of exercise)	• Panic symptoms (e.g., shortness of breath) may be misinterpreted as related cancer and its treatment • Efforts to prevent breathlessness and autonomic arousal may result in avoidance of physical activity and deconditioning
Agoraphobia	• Persistent fear of two or more of the following situations: public transportation, open spaces, enclosed spaces, crowds, and being away from home alone • Situations are feared or avoided due to thoughts that escape may be difficult or help may not be available	• Fear of leaving home or traveling may interfere with attending medical appointments • Additional strain may be placed on social supports to help with transportation

Social Anxiety Disorder	• Persistent fear of social situations and potential negative evaluation by others • Social situations almost always trigger anxiety and are avoided or endured with extreme fear	• Fear of embarrassment or humiliation may inhibit patient advocating for self and communicating with cancer care providers • Cancer-related body disfigurement or changes in physical appearance due to treatment may worsen social anxiety
Substance/ Medication-Induced Anxiety Disorder	• Anxiety or panic symptoms result from substance intoxication or withdrawal or medication side effects • Symptoms are neither explained by another anxiety disorder nor due to delirium	• Withdrawal from nicotine, alcohol, sedatives, and opioids may induce anxiety • Medications commonly used in cancer care that may also induce or mimic anxiety include corticosteroids, antiemetics, interferons, stimulants, antipsychotics, and anticholinergics
Anxiety Disorder Due to Another Medical Condition	• Anxiety or panic symptoms result directly from pathophysiological consequences of another medical condition • Symptoms are neither explained by another mental disorder nor due to delirium	• Common medical conditions in cancer associated with causing or worsening anxiety symptoms include uncontrolled pain, hypercalcemia, CNS tumors, seizures, carcinoid syndrome, heart failure, chronic lung disease, pulmonary effusions or embolism, and sepsis

Note. DSM-5 = Diagnostic and Statistical Manual of Mental Disorders (5th ed.; Washington, DC: American Psychiatric Association; 2013); CNS = central nervous system.

Adapted with permission from JC Holland et al., eds., *Psycho-Oncology*. 3rd ed. Oxford: Oxford University Press; 2015.

anticholinergic drugs (e.g., diphenhydramine, benztropine), and drug withdrawal (e.g., benzodiazepine, alcohol, narcotic medications) should be considered on the differential diagnosis of anxiety.
- Screening for akathisia. Older antiemetics (e.g., prochlorperazine, metoclopramide, promethazine) and antipsychotic medications (e.g., olanzapine, risperidone, haloperidol) may cause akathisia, which is an internal sense of severe anxiety and restlessness associated with motor agitation.

The assessment of distress or anxiety should consider predisposing or contributing factors (i.e., pretest probability) for encountering pathologic anxiety (see Figure 1.1 for overall guidance and summary).

Risk for anxiety is increased if there is a history of anxiety or trauma, avoidant coping style, social isolation, or certain life roles (e.g., caregiver); in certain cancer-related situations (e.g., during treatment/procedures, uncertain disease course, cardiac/pulmonary/central nervous system comorbidities); and with comorbid symptom burden (e.g., depression, insomnia, fatigue, pain) or if dissociative symptoms were present at the time of diagnosis. Premorbid anxiety is the greatest predictor for comorbid anxiety recurrence during the first year following diagnosis.

Screening questionnaires for anxiety specifically vary, from a single-item question "How anxious have you felt this week?" to brief questionnaires, of which the HADS and the General Anxiety Disorder 7-item scale (GAD 7) have accumulated the most psychometric data. Other instruments may screen for specific disorders such as panic or PTSD.

Treatment

The treatment of anxiety disorders in patients with cancer includes a range of pharmacologic, psychosocial, and psycho-educational interventions. The clinical management of anxiety disorders should be directed toward the specifically diagnosed anxiety disorder and is similar to treatment in the general population.

Psychotherapy. Psychosocial interventions consist of education and psychotherapy (CBT and supportive-expressive), stress management, and supportive counseling. CBT therapies are goal-oriented and focus on restructuring thinking patterns and behaviors, while supportive-expressive therapies offer a nondirective approach that allows patients to process their cancer-related experiences. Mind-body approaches may be helpful to ameliorate anxiety symptoms. Patients should be encouraged to utilize other available sources (e.g., chaplain, local cancer organizations).

Psychotropic medication. Pharmacologic interventions in cancer should be guided by the anxiety diagnosis, side-effect profile of the drug, symptom severity, and patient preference. See chapter 5 for details about psychotropic medication. In panic disorder, antidepressant medications should be started at recommended low doses or even lower to ensure tolerability. Attention should be given to titrating the psychotropic medication to achieve the desired beneficial effect. Patients should be maintained on antidepressant medication for at least two to four weeks unless they are not tolerating the side effects. For generalized anxiety disorder, therapeutic trials of anxiolytic medications do not last as long since their benefit is seen within a couple of doses. Certain antipsychotic medications (e.g., olanzapine) are now more commonly used in oncology settings to alleviate anxiety or for chemotherapy-induced nausea or hiccups. Indications for the use of psychotropic medication in oncology extends beyond mood disorders to cancer-related fatigue, anorexia and weight loss, hot flashes, delirium, sleep disturbances, nausea, and chemotherapy-induced neuropathy. There are few data about the relative or additive effects of pharmacology to psychosocial interventions in the cancer setting.

Benzodiazepines may play a useful role in helping the anxious cancer patient. However, all benzodiazepines have potential side effects of sedation, dizziness, incoordination, and potential for tolerance and abuse or dependence. The shortest acting benzodiazepine (alprazolam), in particular, can cause rebound anxiety and has a higher risk of abuse and dependence. Its use should be limited to specific indications (e.g., one-time administration for procedures, to abort a panic in panic disorder). All benzodiazepines may cause bradycardia and respiratory depression (particularly with diazepam and lorazepam), drug–drug interactions (e.g., alprazolam and triazolam), impaired memory and disorientation, rebound anxiety, and the potential for withdrawal symptoms. A clear indication and monitoring plan should be prescribed for the patient, and these medications should be reserved for moderate to severe symptoms.

Hypnotics may be prescribed for short-term insomnia after a detailed history of sleep hygiene, depression, anxiety, and substance use are reviewed and sleep hygiene education, relaxation training, and other nonpharmacological approaches have been attempted. Hypnotics that act on the GABAergic system are preferred such as zolpidem or zaleplon.

Specific disorders. Most cancer-related anxiety therapies take a generalist approach, but specific anxiety disorders should be managed by more directed approaches. For example, comorbid panic disorder may be treated using systematic desensitization (i.e., type of CBT) and/or FDA-approved medications: fluoxetine, paroxetine, sertraline, and/or the SNRI venlafaxine. Generalized anxiety disorder treatment may utilize various psychotherapies and/or the commonly used antidepressants fluoxetine, paroxetine, escitalopram, sertraline, venlafaxine, imipramine, and duloxetine. PTSD should be treated with the FDA-approved agents sertraline and/or paroxetine.

Oncology teams should utilize appropriate referrals for specialized supportive care (e.g., pastoral care, palliative care, social work) when necessary. Psycho-oncologists must have knowledge of psychiatric medication use in oncology, since up to 50% of patients will take a psychiatric medication (e.g., anxiolytic, hypnotic, antidepressant) during the course of their illness. Consulting teams may put together a complete psychosocial plan to comprehensively address the patient's problems. Mental health professionals should manage most severe anxiety disorders.

Case Study

Anxiety Disorder Management

Mrs. S has always described herself as an anxious person. Three years ago she was diagnosed with de novo metastatic breast cancer and has done very well on selective estrogen receptor modulators. After switching medications a few times, she was able to tolerate the hot flashes and some of the achy joint stiffness. Of late, she reports multiple relationship difficulties that have led to an employment demotion and less support from her husband and family. Upon hearing this news, the oncologist probes a little deeper into the situation and finds that she has been avoiding going to work since she had a panic attack on her way to work three months ago and several have recurred since. She did want to discuss this with her oncology team because she was embarrassed and did not want the oncology team to be distracted from treating her cancer. After being reassured by her oncologist about the importance of treating anxiety that is impairing her ability to function in her life, she agrees to meet with a mental health professional about her panic attacks. After receiving information about the diagnosis, starting psychotherapy, and venlafaxine (also used to treat hot flashes), she reports that she is now able to go to work and has improved her relationships at home as well.

Professional Issues and Service Implementation

The psycho-oncologist can help all of the oncology treatment team to better understand an anxious patient by recording an overview in the medical chart of who this person is, what factors have contributed developmentally to his or her anxious disposition, and what strategies may help the individual to cope optimally with the illness. Extra effort may be needed to educate the patient about his or her illness and its treatment, manage side effects, limit bodily hypervigilance, and sustain hope and optimism and thus optimize quality of life. The multidisciplinary team needs to use a consistent approach to be helpful, avoiding mixed messages and ensuring effective communication between its members.

The common ethical dilemmas that arise in very anxious patients include

- Treatment decisions, where excessive worry about treatment side effects may lead a patient to consider foregoing curative treatments.
- Whether patients truly understand the risks of the side effects they are worried about.
- Discordance of views between patients or family members and the treating physician or team (e.g., regarding consent to treatment or withdrawal of active anticancer treatments).

Difficult situations for treating professionals should be brought to the ethics committee at the local hospital. Ethical issues tend to resolve themselves when perspectives are obtained from multiple disciplines.

The medical provider who is administering treatment has a legal responsibility to deliver care as dictated by "standard of care" practices. This agreement may be tacit and not explicit, and the medical professional should always follow through to either provide the necessary care or help to facilitate the care that should be provided.

Conclusion

The recognition and management of distress and anxiety are playing a larger role than ever in providing quality cancer care. New ways to incorporate distress screening and the treatments of anxiety and adjustment disorders into the cancer continuum should be forthcoming. NCCN guideline recommendations should be followed by oncology practices, and psycho-oncology teams should provide expert consultative care for the myriad of comorbidly presenting disorders in cancer. The most important test continues to be a thorough history, with supporting collateral information from the patient's primary caregiver, family, friends, neighbors, and/or emergency medical personnel or police. The efficacy of available treatments comes from the ability to improve communication with patients, psychoeducation, reduction of stigma, repeat assessments, and collaborations with other cancer-treating professionals.

References

1. Mitchell AJ, Chan M, Bhatti H, et al. Prevalence of depression, anxiety, and adjustment disorder in oncological, haematological, and palliative-care settings: a meta-analysis of 94 interview-based studies. *Lancet Oncol.* 2011;12(2):160–174.

2. Mitchell AJ. Pooled results from 38 analyses of the accuracy of distress thermometer and other ultra-short methods of detecting cancer-related mood disorders. *J Clin Oncol.* 2007;25(29):4670–4681.

3. Mehnert A, Brahler E, Faller H, et al. Four-week prevalence of mental disorders in patients with cancer across major tumor entities. *J Clin Oncol.* 2014;32(31):3540–3546.

4. Weisman AD, Worden JW. The existential plight in cancer: significance of the first 100 days. *Int J Psychiatry Med.* 1976;7(1):1–15.

5. Cancer care for the whole patient: meeting psychosocial health needs [press release]. Washington, DC: National Academies Press; 2008.

6. Brintzenhofe-Szoc KM, Levin TT, Li Y, Kissane DW, Zabora JR. Mixed anxiety/depression symptoms in a large cancer cohort: prevalence by cancer type. *Psychosomatics.* 2009;50(4):383–391.

7. Miovic M, Block S. Psychiatric disorders in advanced cancer. *Cancer.* 2007;110(8):1665–1676.

8. Delgado-Guay M, Parsons HA, Li Z, Palmer JL, Bruera E. Symptom distress in advanced cancer patients with anxiety and depression in the palliative care setting. *Support Care Cancer.* 2009;17(5):573–579.

9. Barbera L, Seow H, Howell D, et al. Symptom burden and performance status in a population-based cohort of ambulatory cancer patients. *Cancer.* 2010;116(24):5767–5776.

10. Kangas M, Henry JL, Bryant RA. The course of psychological disorders in the 1st year after cancer diagnosis. *J Consult Clin Psychol.* 2005;73(4):763–768.

Further Reading

Grassi L, Riba M, eds. *Clinical Psycho-Oncology: An International Perspective.* Chichester, UK: Wiley-Blackwell; 2012.

This textbook is recommended for its international and cultural perspectives.

Holland J, Breitbart WS, Jacobsen PB, Loscalzo MJ, McCorkle R, Butow PN, eds. *Psycho-oncology.* 3rd ed. Oxford, New York: Oxford University Press; 2012.

This textbook is recommended for its detailed summary of information that provides more depth about distress, adjustment disorder, and anxiety disorders in the cancer context.

Watson M, Kissane D, eds. *Handbook of Psychotherapy in Cancer Care.* Chichester, UK: Wiley-Blackwell; 2011.

This handbook focuses on strategies and techniques used in psychotherapy with patients with cancer and their families.

Chapter Quiz

Questions

1. Distress became an official psychiatric diagnosis in 1997.
   A. True
   B. False

2. Types of adjustment disorders include which of the following?
   A. With melancholia and alexithymia
   B. With anxiety
   C. With depressed mood
   D. With sardonic features
   E. With mixed anxiety and depressed mood

3. There is a strong association between certain cancer types that predispose to distress and anxiety.
   A. True
   B. False

4. Adjustment disorders must be diagnosed within six months of the related stressor.
   A. True
   B. False

5. Which of the following anxiety disorders is most common in the cancer setting?
   A. Generalized anxiety disorder
   B. Panic disorder
   C. Posttraumatic stress disorder
   D. Obsessive compulsive disorder
   E. Adjustment disorder with anxiety
   F. Anxiety due to general medical condition

Chapter 2

Depression in Cancer Care

Daisuke Fujisawa and Yosuke Uchitomi

Learning Objectives

After reading this chapter, the clinician will be able to
1. Understand the signs and symptoms of depression in clinical practice.
2. Conduct a comprehensive assessment, including making differential diagnoses and assessing the psychosocial needs of patients.
3. Understand the basic principles of treatment, including use of psychotropic medication and psychotherapy.
4. Make a referral to a specialist when appropriate.

Background Evidence

A recent meta-analysis[1] reveals the prevalence of major depression among cancer patients according to stringent criteria as 16.3% (13.4%–19.5%). Another 19.2% (9.1%–31.9%) of cancer patients suffer from minor depression (a milder type of depression, which may impair functioning and quality of life of patients). These rates are at least three times as high as those found in the general population.[2] These numbers increase further when depression "caseness" is defined as patients who score above a certain cutoff value on a depression screening instrument.

Depression not only causes suffering to patients, but it also impairs patients' well-being in many ways. Even a mild level of depression can cause significant decrements in quality of life, which is comparable to decrements due to major physical symptom burdens and decreased performance status.[3] In many studies, depression is associated with shorter survival in cancer patients, due to both death by cancer and death by other causes.[4,5] Lower survival of patients with depression is partly explained by poorer adherence to cancer treatment,[6] poorer self-care (e.g., unfavorable lifestyle such as decreased level of physical exercise, higher alcohol consumption, or inappropriate diet), and proneness to medical decisions that may shorten life (e.g., receiving chemotherapy at the very end of life, which can do more harm than good regarding survival). There is some evidence that depression decreases immune function, although its relationship with cancer prognosis remains unclear.[7] In clinical management, patients with depression tend to stay longer in hospitals. Depression often increases sensitivity to and monitoring of physical sensations and thereby may increase pain. Depression is a large contributor to the wish for hastened death (e.g., suicide, physician-assisted suicide, euthanasia, and rejection of proper treatment).

Depression is frequently underrecognized and undertreated. Patients with cancer are not an exception. Severe depression is more likely to be underrecognized, since patients with severe depression tend to express their emotions less than those with milder depression. Therefore, routine screening is considered vital in oncology practice.[8]

Presenting Problems

Key Symptoms and Signs

Depression is a syndrome characterized by depressed mood and anhedonia. It is a spectrum of symptoms, where normal sadness or grief occurs at the milder end and major depression at the opposite (more severe) end. Minor or subthreshold depression lies in the middle.

Major depression is a diagnostic category characterized by five or more (out of nine) depressive symptoms present for most of the day for at least two weeks. At least one of those five symptoms must be depressed mood or anhedonia (decreased interest or diminished sense of pleasure). The other symptoms include decreased energy, remarkable change in appetite (decrease or increase of appetite, which can be allied with change in body weight), sleep disturbance (either insomnia or hypersomnia), psychomotor agitation or retardation (i.e., patients may objectively look irritable or slow in actions), feelings of worthlessness or guilt, difficulty concentrating, and suicidal ideation (see Box 2.1).

Box 2.1 Diagnosis of Major Depression

1. Depressed mood
2. Anhedonia (lack of interest or pleasure in almost all activities)
3. Sleep disorder (insomnia or hypersomnia)
4. Appetite loss, weight loss; appetite gain, weight gain
5. Fatigue or loss of energy
6. Psychomotor retardation (a patient looks slow in actions or responses) or agitation (a patient looks irritable and hasty)
7. Trouble concentrating or trouble making decisions
8. Low self-esteem or feelings of guilt
9. Recurrent thoughts of death or suicidal ideation

Five of these symptoms are required to make the diagnosis of depression and must include depressed mood and/or anhedonia.

Note: The symptoms must have been present most of the day, nearly every day for at least two weeks. The symptoms cannot be explained by other physical or psychiatric problems.

(Abstracted from American Psychiatric Association. *Diagnostic and Statistical Manual of Mental Disorders*, 5th ed. Washington, DC: American Psychiatric Association, 2013).

A patient is diagnosed as having minor (or subthreshold) depression when two to four of these symptoms are present for at least two weeks. A state whereby three to four depressive symptoms are present continuously for at least two years is called dysthymia (chronic depression).

The diagnostic term *adjustment disorder* is often used for milder forms of depression. It refers to a state of moderate to marked distress that is greater than expected from exposure to a stressor and may present with depressive symptoms. However, difficulty in defining normative distress in the context of cancer raises questions about its diagnostic validity. Differentiation between major or minor depression and adjustment disorder is often ambiguous. *The rule of thumb is that, although life stressors may seem to provide "good reasons" for sadness, the diagnosis of depression should not be withheld if a patient meets the criteria for major/minor depression.* Usually, patients with more severe and more pervasive symptoms have depression rather than a nonpathological reaction to stressful events. These symptoms include loss of emotional reactivity to good news (e.g., a patient who does not feel joy in response to hospital visits of close family), irrational sense of self-guilt (e.g., patients who believe it is their fault they have cancer), and suicidal thoughts with plans.

Although minor depression is described as a milder form of depression, it is associated with significant impairment of quality of life and can be critical, especially among vulnerable populations such as older people or those with poor socioeconomic status. A family history of psychiatric illness and the presence of chronic medical illness are risk factors for conversion from minor to major depression.

Key Problems Associated with Development of Depression

Depression can occur in patients with any type of cancer and at any stage of illness. Key risk factors for depression include

- advanced illness
- past history of depression
- other psychiatric disorders
- higher symptom burden
- more frequent unmet needs

Key consequences of depression include

- reduced quality of life and poorer fitness
- poor adherence to medication and anticancer treatment
- reduced overall survival
- poorer health associated with other illnesses
- risk of reduced social support

Diagnosis and Assessment

Careful evaluation of past psychiatric history and current physical and psychosocial problems are essential.

Diagnosis

Clinical interview. The diagnosis of depression is made by clinical interview. Formally, clinicians may refer to a manual of the Structured Clinical Interview for the *Diagnostic and Statistical Manual of Mental Disorders*. In actual clinical practice, clinicians simply ask whether a patient has each symptom of depression.

- Depressed mood

    "How has your mood been the last few weeks?"

    "Have you been feeling sad, blue, or down in the last few weeks?"

- Anhedonia

    "What do you enjoy doing these days?"

    "Have you lost interest or pleasure in what you used to enjoy doing?"

The US Preventive Services Task Force recommends a straightforward, two-item screening for major depression that has been proven to be as effective as longer screening instruments. A positive answer to either of these two questions should prompt clinicians to perform a full diagnostic assessment of major depression:

- "Over the past two weeks, have you ever felt down, depressed, or hopeless?"
- "Over the past two weeks, have you felt little interest or pleasure doing things?"

Self-administered instruments. Self-administered instruments can be good diagnostic aids for clinicians, although they are not substitutes for clinical interviews. Screening instruments for depression that are widely used in oncology settings include, but are not limited to, the following:

- Hospital Anxiety and Depression Scale (HADS)

    The HADS is the most widely used measure in oncology settings. Its positive features include its brevity and its ability to perform adequately across different stages of cancer. Because it does not include somatic symptoms, it eliminates the influence of physical conditions. The most commonly used threshold to define depression is a subscale score of 8 or above, although variability in recommended cutoff scores (ranging from 4 to 11) has been reported and is considered a limitation of the scale.

- Patient Health Questionnaire (PHQ-9)

    Although less well-studied in oncology settings compared with the HADS, the PHQ was initially developed for use in primary care settings, including patients with chronic medical illness. A score of 10 or higher has been demonstrated to have 88% sensitivity and 88% specificity for the diagnosis of major depression. Some items can be problematic because they may be influenced by symptoms of cancer and cancer treatment. The PHQ-9 can helpfully demonstrate change in depressive symptoms following treatment of the illness.

- Beck Depression Inventory (BDI)

    The classic BDI and its variations (the BDI-II and the BDI-Short Form [BDI-SF]) are often considered the "gold standard" scales for depression. The advantages of the scale include the broad rather than narrow face validity of its items, its generalizability across cancer types and stages, and its strong reliability and validity. Its limitations include the length (21 items), which can reduce acceptability, and inclusion of somatic symptoms; the BDI-SF removes physical symptoms and has obvious benefits in oncology practice.

Monitoring progress

One of the most significant primary care errors in managing depression is failure to monitor the treatment progress and not titrating the antidepressant dose upward once the medication is commenced. Regular administration of self-report questionnaires can help clinicians evaluate patients' responses to treatment of depression. The questionnaires listed here can also be used for monitoring.

Factors that contribute to misdiagnosis or inappropriate care

Devastating physical consequences from cancer and its treatment can mimic depressive symptoms. For example, poor appetite, weight loss, and fatigue can be symptoms due to cancer (and cancer treatments) or depression. These are differentiated by assessing the presence of depressive mood or anhedonia.

Exemplary diagnostic questions include the following:

- "Do you feel depressed all the time? Or do you feel better when your physical symptoms are relatively better?" (If a patient replies "yes" to the latter question, he or she probably does not have a depressive mood symptom.)
- "Are you motivated to do something if your physical symptoms are relieved?" (If a patient replies "yes," he or she is probably not anhedonic.)
- The rule of thumb is to diagnose a patient as depressed unless there is clear evidence that his or her depressive symptoms come from physical issues in order to avoid missing the chance to help the patient recover from depression (inclusive approach).

Case Study

A 60-year-old male with a diagnosis of multiple myeloma is referred to a psycho-oncologist. The reason for referral is his unwillingness to participate in rehabilitation and prominent anxiety, which prevents his hospital discharge. Close interview reveals persistent depressive mood, lack of appetite, poor sleep, and excessive fatigue that cannot be well explained by his physical condition, as well as lack of motivation toward everything, not just rehabilitation. The patient is diagnosed as having major depression, and mirtazapine 15 mg (before sleep) is started. His sleep improves immediately, and his appetite begins to pick up within three days. Although the patient's mood improves a bit, he is hesitant to move out of his bed partly because of fatigue. Based on the principles of behavioral activation (see later sections for detail), the psychiatrist encourages the patient to gradually increase his activity level. With collaboration of the psychiatrist, psychologist, physiotherapist, nurses, the patient, and his family, the treatment team creates an activity schedule, which initially includes minimal activities and later increased activities. Also, elaborate conversations with the patient reveal that his unwillingness to move comes from the fear of falling and fear of breaking his bones, which he believes are seriously affected by his multiple myeloma. Also, he believes that he will not recover from his multiple myeloma because he is feeling very unwell. Followed by reassurance from the treating physician, the psychologist explains the concept of cognitive biases (see Table 2.3) and facilitates cognitive reframing (see later sections for detail). The patient becomes more active after a week and starts participating in rehabilitation. Although his anxiety about discharge is observable, the primary care team coordinates his discharge, after a "trial" of an overnight stay at home, which helps reassure him about his recovery.

Investigations for Key Differential Diagnosis

Key Differentials

Physical conditions

- Unsolved physical distress (e.g., pain, nausea)
- Endocrine dysfunction (e.g., hyperthyroidism, hypothyroidism, adrenal insufficiency) such as those caused by either surgical resection, radiation therapy, or cancer metastases.
- Anemia
- Nutritional deficits/imbalance such as vitamin deficiency (vitamin B3 [nicotinic acid, niacin], vitamin B12, folate, vitamin C)
- Electrolyte imbalance (sodium, potassium, calcium, magnesium)
- Cancer-related fatigue (see Table 2.1)
- Other exhausting physical conditions, such as cardiac dysfunction, hepatic dysfunction, infection, pulmonary dysfunction

Medications (side effects)

- Steroids, interferon, beta-adrenergic blockers
- Late effect of anticancer agents ("chemobrain")

Organic brain disorders

- Brain tumor or metastasis, especially frontal lobe apathy
- Meningitis carcinomatosa, or leptomeningeal disease
- Paraneoplastic syndrome, with serum and cerebrospinal fluid autoimmune antibodies

Table 2.1 Distinguishing Fatigue from Depression	
Fatigue	Patients usually are able to derive some pleasure from activities that they normally find enjoyable
	Late afternoon is the most difficult time of the day
Depression	Patients are unable to experience pleasure from experiences that they usually enjoy
	Morning is the most difficult time of the day
	Past history and/or family history of major depression may increase the likelihood of developing an episode of depression. In cases of uncertainty, an empiric trial of antidepressant therapy may be indicated in order not to let a possible case of depression go untreated
Note: Fatigue and depression may be concurrent.	

Neurological disorders
- Parkinson syndrome, multiple sclerosis, HIV encephalopathy, cerebrovascular diseases

Changed mental status
- Minimal consciousness disturbance, including delirium (especially hypoactive delirium)
- Dementia (although depression can be comorbid with dementia)

Other psychiatric/psychological states
- Alcohol/substance abuse (chronic alcohol abuse can cause depressive symptoms, which can be alleviated by abstinence)
- Normal grief (normal psychological reaction to stress)
- Demoralization syndrome (see chapter 3)

Essential Tests
- Neuroimaging: CAT scan, MRI (Gd-enhancement to detect subtle brain metastasis and meningitis carcinomatosa), PET
- Laboratory tests: to exclude anemia (Hb, Ht), electrolyte disturbance (Na, K, Ca, Mg), hypoglycaemia (Glu), endocrine disorders (thyroid tests [TSH, fT3, fT4], ACTH, cortisol), and liver function tests if metastatic liver disease
- Electroencephalogram (EEG): if consciousness disturbance is hard to rule out.

Further Assessments
Depression can be masked, and diagnosis and evaluation of depression cannot occur without clinical interviews; however, some patients, especially older patients and those with severe depressive symptoms, may not explicitly admit to lowered mood, which can make the assessment difficult. The following objective appearance and behaviors of patients may be signs of depression.
- Social withdrawal
- Not participating in medical care
- Diminished positive emotional reactions (e.g., not able to be cheered up, does not smile, no response to good news or funny situations)
- Demeanor showing reduced facial reactivity and slowed thinking

Clinical Management

Treatment of depression should not target depressive symptoms only but should also address all kinds of disease-related and psychosocial factors that contribute to the emergence of depression. These include physical symptoms such as pain, poor test results or prognosis, problematic relationships with medical providers, lack of social support, and other psychosocial issues.

Referral
Routine screening for depression is recommended. Once the presence of depressive symptoms is suspected, clinicians should conduct a more

comprehensive assessment for depression based on the diagnostic criteria and improve their understanding of the whole person and his or her family. Addressing any bio- or psychosocial problems and concerns is required, regardless of whether the patient is diagnosed as depressed. Depression should be treated based on the level of severity. Routine screening is necessary, especially at critical time points of cancer treatment (e.g., when cancer progression is imminent, during transition from one treatment modality to another; see Figure 2.1).

Comprehensive assessment and support should be provided to every patient. Use of screening tools that comprehensively assess symptoms and functions, such as the Edmonton Symptom Assessment Scale or the MD Anderson Symptom Inventory may be useful.

Psychotherapy (psychological treatment) is indicated at all levels of depression severity. Pharmacotherapy is an option for mild to moderate depression and is a requirement for severe depression (see chapter 5). All treatments should be tailored based on patients' preference, their physical condition, and access to care.

Good communication between clinicians and patients is fundamental to preventing and alleviating depression. For example, providing communication-skill training to oncologists can result in a decrease in psychological distress among their patients.[9] Proactive, detailed assessment and addressing patients' needs and concerns are important components of psychosocial care. In addition, provision of palliative care integrated into routine oncology practice from an earlier stage of treatment for advanced lung cancer patients has been shown to alleviate depression without increasing referral to mental-health specialists.[10]

Pharmacological Options

General principles

Here we provide broad principles regarding and reasons for selecting specific psychotropic medications in the treatment of depression. For detailed information, see chapter 5.

The following classes of psychotropics may be used in the care of depression. Many antidepressants are metabolized by CYP 450. Clinicians should be watchful for potential interactions with other medications in use.

All benzodiazepine anxiolytics are metabolized in the liver and have active metabolites, except for lorazepam, which is metabolized through glucuronidation without active metabolites, therefore it is relatively safely used for patients with liver dysfunction. See chapter 5 for details.

Antidepressants. Antidepressants are the key drugs for treating depression. However, because of their gradual action (usually they take a few weeks before they become effective), other classes of psychotropics (psychostimulants, anxiolytics, or neuroleptics) may be preferred in some situations (e.g., a patient with extremely severe depression who needs urgent relief or a patient with extremely poor prognosis who cannot wait for weeks).

Anxiolytics

(a) Anxiolytics, usually benzodiazepines ("minor tranquilizers"), may be used as adjunctive medication to antidepressants to alleviate distress,

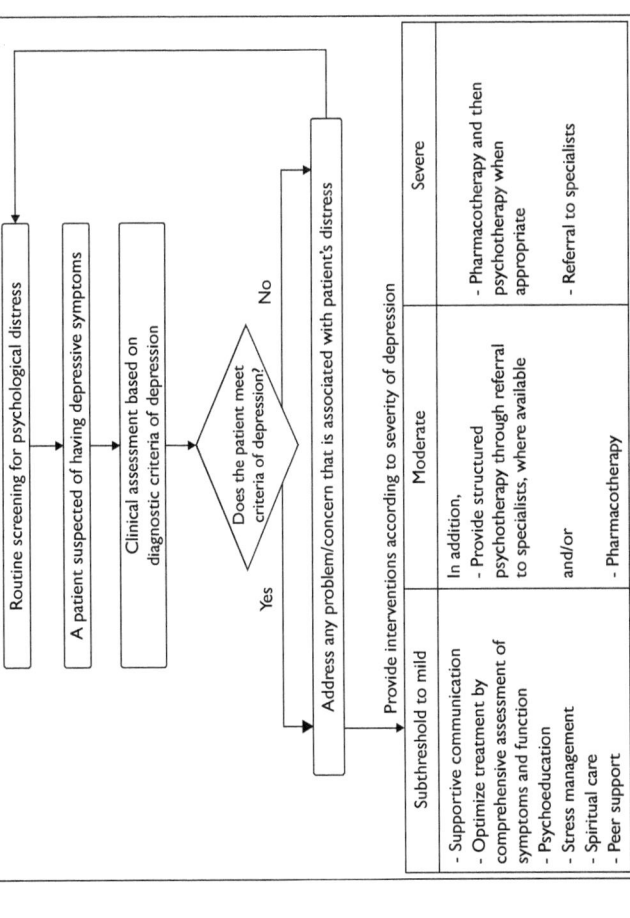

Figure 2.1. Overall management algorithm for distress and anxiety in cancer care. Adapted with permission from the NCCN guidelines.

anxiety, and/or agitation of depressed patients. Its quick effect is considered favorable by patients and clinicians, although its effectiveness for depression in the long term (> four weeks) has not been proven. Caution is necessary as benzodiazepines may induce delirium in vulnerable patients such as older patients or those with advanced illness.

(b) Buspiron is a drug that has anxiolytic effects. In contrast to benzodiazepines, tolerability of buspiron is high (i.e., its adverse effects are mild), despite its effectiveness as a sole agent in treating depression being limited. Its adjunctive use with selective serotonin reuptake inhibitors (SSRIs) is helpful.

Hypnotics. Hypnotics (usually benzodiazepines) are helpful for patients who have trouble sleeping. The same cautions apply as those for anxiolytics (see previous section).

Neuroleptics: (Antipsychotics or "Major tranquilizers"). Neuroleptics are used either as an augmentation therapy for depression or as an alternative for anxiolytics, especially for patients with severe symptoms that cannot be alleviated by benzodiazepines or for patients at risk of adverse effects of benzodiazepines including dependence. The more extended use of neuroleptics does not cause addiction as it does for benzodiazepines. Some antipsychotics (e.g., quetiapine, aripiprazole) themselves have antidepressant effects.

Side effects
Antidepressants
SSRIs/SNRIs

- Nausea/emesis, which occurs at the beginning of administration. Clinicians should inform patients that nausea/emesis may occur as an adverse effect but usually disappears within a few days. Postcibal administration (e.g., taken after breakfast) reduces the risk of nausea. Antiemetic drugs (e.g., mosapride, metoclopramide) can be prescribed for these side effects.
- Sleep disturbance (either insomnia or hypersomnia).
- Sexual dysfunction, which is often underreported by patients. This should be mentioned in advance by clinicians. Sexual dysfunction can also be a part of depressive symptoms that can be resolved as depression resolves.
- Bleeding diatheses. Since serotonin is one of the chemotactic factors associated with platelet aggregation, administration of SSRIs can increase the risk of bleeding, especially for the patients who are already taking NSAIDs or other antiplatelet medications.
- Syndrome of inappropriate antidiuretic hormone secretion (SIADH). Antidepressants, especially SSRIs, serotonin–norepinephrine reuptake inhibitors (SNRIs), and tricyclics, can cause SIADH, whereby water retention causes euvolemic hyponatremia.
- "Activation syndrome." In a small group of individuals, SSRIs and SNRIs may cause irritability, agitation, or dysphoria at the beginning of administration. This can be alleviated by decreasing the dose, switching medicine, or concurrently using benzodiazepines.

- "Withdrawal syndrome." Abrupt stopping of an SSRI or SNRI can present with severe dizziness, fatigue, and dysphoria, arising from re-adaptation of receptors. High doses of SSRIs/SNRIs should be tapered rather than be stopped abruptly. Readministration of the drug alleviates those symptoms.

Mirtazapine
- Sleepiness.
- Increased appetite. In contrast to SSRIs/SNRIs, mirtazapine usually does not cause nausea/emesis and can be helpful for cancer patients who suffer from appetite loss not only due to depression but also due to cancer progression and cancer treatment.

Tricyclics
- Tricyclic antidepressants (TCAs) are older-generation antidepressants that generally have more frequent adverse effects and lower tolerability. Since their effectiveness is not significantly different from those of newer generation antidepressants (e.g., SSRIs/SNRIs, mirtazapine, bupropion), TCAs are seldom used as a first-line antidepressant. Some TCAs may be used because of strong analgesic effects.
- Anticholinergic effects, especially for cancer patients.

Anxiolytics: Benzodiazepines or "minor tranquilizers."
- Sleepiness, fatigue, and decreased concentration, which can impair daily functioning.
- Dizziness and muscle weakness (due to its muscle-relaxant effect), which can create a risk of falls.
- Decreased wakefulness, which can lead to delirium.

Note that these side effects are usually reversible and would cease once the drug is discontinued.

Light Therapy

Light therapy is applied for patients with seasonal affective disorder. This disorder is characterized by recurrent depressive episodes that occur during autumn and winter, alternating with nondepressive episodes during spring and summer. Light therapy, which involves exposing patients to special equipment that produces bright white light, is proven to prevent and improve development of depression during the winter.

Electroconvulsive Therapy

Electroconvulsive therapy (ECT) is a treatment of choice for patients with depression refractory to pharmacotherapy, patients with psychotic depression, and for some patients who are acutely suicidal. New methods of administration of ECT (modified-ECT [m-ECT]) have been proven safe and can be even safer than antidepressants. Therefore, m-ECT is also indicated for vulnerable populations such as the elderly, who cannot be provided with standard pharmacotherapy due to adverse effects.

Psychological Treatments (Psychotherapy)

There is robust evidence supporting psychological treatments for patients with cancer, and a variety of techniques and methods have been developed and examined for their effectiveness in the psychological care of cancer patients (see Table 2.2).

General principles

Before implementing a psychotherapeutic strategy, it is important to develop a formulation and to consider whether the patient is eligible for psychotherapy, what type of psychotherapy is most suitable, and what the patient's preferences are regarding treatment approach.

Generally, implementation of psychotherapy requires that patients are highly motivated and that symptoms of clinical depression do not represent a barrier to patients' abilities to use talking therapies. Use of cognitive behavioral therapy (CBT) is indicated for patients with physical health problems based on accumulated evidence from the UK National Institute for Health and Care Excellence (NICE Guidelines). Patients with advanced cancers

Table 2.2 Type of Psychotherapies

Term	Description
Counseling	A generic term to describe supportive psychosocial care provided by a qualified professional.
Psychoeducation	Provision of information designed to increase knowledge, reduce uncertainty, and thereby enhance psychological well-being.
Relaxation training and mindfulness therapies	Teaching skills to release physical or mental tension using various methods, including meditation, progressive muscle relaxation, breathing techniques, or use of guided mental imagery. Mindfulness-based therapies developed from a different origin but can be used as a part of stress-reduction techniques.
Problem-solving therapy	A therapy that focuses on generating solutions to identified problems through a structured, step-by-step approach.
Cognitive behavioral therapy	A therapy that focuses on identifying and challenging maladaptive thoughts and behaviors, thereby eliciting adaptive, more functional thoughts and behaviors. Behavioral activation is part of cognitive behavioral therapy technique, which is sometimes provided as stand-alone form.
Interpersonal therapy	A therapy that focuses on problems within interpersonal interactions and relationships, emphasizing areas such as grief, role transitions, disputes, or interpersonal deficits.
Supportive-expressive therapy	A therapy that focuses on the communication and processing of subjective experience and on the joint creation of meaning. Many psychotherapies can be classified under this category, including psychodynamic therapy, meaning-centered therapy, dignity therapy, and CALM therapy.

may also benefit from supportive-expressive therapies, including meaning-centered psychotherapy, mindfulness-based cognitive therapy, dignity therapy, and CALM (Managing Cancer and Living Meaningfully) therapy.

Cognitive behavioral therapy

Theoretical background. Cognitive behavioral therapy (CBT), or cognitive therapy, is a structured psychotherapy based on the hypothesis that one's emotional and somatic responses (mood and physical symptoms) are determined by how one perceives a situation, rather than the situation itself. A triggering situation leads to an "automatic negative thought," which generates a response that can be emotional (e.g., depression), behavioral (e.g., withdrawal), or physical (e.g., fatigue, breathlessness).

Cognitive reframing. People with marked depression or anxiety can have inflexible overgeneralized thoughts ("cognitive bias"). Identifying and reframing these dysfunctional (maladaptive) automatic thoughts into more functional (realistic or adaptive) is an important component of CBT. In the process of reframing, therapists educate patients about typical cognitive biases (some examples are listed in Table 2.3) and encourage them to challenge these

Table 2.3 Common Cognitive Biases

Cognitive Biases	Examples	More Adaptive Response upon Reframing
All-or-none thinking	If I can't be cured, there is no meaning of doing anything.	Even if my cancer is not curable, treatment can prolong my life for a certain period and may improve my quality of life.
Overgeneralization	This pain killer was not effective. Drugs are of no use!	The nurse told me that there are many kinds of drugs. Try and see which medicine suits me.
Magnification/ minimization	Chemotherapy brings me fatigue and does me no good.	Chemotherapy does cause fatigue, but it also brings a curative effect for cancer.
Mind-reading	My husband comes home late these days. He is fed up with life with me having cancer.	My husband comes home late these days. I should ask him how he feels.
"Should" thinking	As an employee, I should work as efficiently as I did before I got cancer.	It is natural that I can't work as efficiently as before cancer treatment. Once treatment is done, I will.
Labeling	I am weak. I live on pain killers.	Use of prescribed drugs has nothing to do with my personality.
Emotional reasoning	I am not feeling well this morning. I am sure today will be a bad day.	I am not feeling well. Let's consider a plan to make today a better day.
Personalization	I deserve my cancer because I didn't eat much vegetables.	There are multiple etiologies for cancer. The influence of my lifestyle is minimal, if any.

biases, verifying their thoughts by looking for evidence (facts) that support or contradict these thoughts.

Behavioral activation. The hypothesis of behavioral activation is that people who are depressed are trapped in the vicious cycle of feeling depressed → loss of energy (motivation) → loss of opportunities of pleasure or feeling of achievement → feeling more depressed. The therapist encourages patients to undertake activities that bring them pleasure or feelings of achievement by encouraging them to develop a schedule of daily activities and monitor mood changes that result from each activity. Although behavioral activation was initially developed as a behavioral component of CBT, it can also be applied as a stand-alone intervention, such as problem-solving therapy.

A fuller explanation of CBT can be found in the *Handbook of Psychotherapy in Cancer Care* (see Further Reading).

Problem-solving therapy

Problem-solving therapy is often described as a simpler or more focused form of CBT and is based on the hypothesis that psychological distress is linked with unsolved problems; therefore, acquisition of efficient problem-solving (or coping) leads to decreased distress.

In the standard problem-solving therapy procedure, the therapist teaches methods of efficacious problem-solving, which is achieved through

- defining the problem.
- brainstorming possible options.
- evaluating potential solutions by weighing advantages and disadvantages of each solution.
- implementing specific solutions.
- evaluating their degree of success.
- fine-tuning them.

Since this is a quite straightforward method, it can be implemented by health professionals who are not specialized in mental health (e.g., primary care nurses) and who have been through a relatively short training.

Relaxation techniques

Relaxation techniques are a widely used method in the field of oncology. Meta-analyses demonstrate its effectiveness for various physical and psychological conditions, including anxiety, depression, breathlessness, and pain, although efficacy appears to be short-lived. Three techniques are typically used: breathing technique; progressive muscle relaxation; and coping self-statements, visualization, or imagery (auto-induction techniques). The evidence indicates this method is more helpful for management of anxiety than depression.

Interpersonal psychotherapy

Interpersonal psychotherapy (IPT) is proven to be as efficacious as CBT, although it has not been well studied in oncology settings. IPT hypothesizes that depression can arise from unsolved issues with people's significant others (i.e., people who are close to them), usually in any of the following four realms: grief, disputes, role transitions, and lack of significant relationships. IPT therapists try to identify the interpersonal problems of the patient and to solve them through various techniques, including cognitive behavioral skills, communication analysis, and training.

Meaning-centered psychotherapy

Meaning-centered psychotherapy is an eight-week manualized intervention that can be delivered in either an individual or a group format. The intervention is influenced by the work of Viktor Frankl's logotherapy and aims to help patients with advanced cancer sustain or enhance a sense of meaning, peace, and purpose in their lives. Each session addresses specific themes related to an exploration of the concepts and sources of meaning (e.g., historical [i.e., legacy], attitudinal, creative, and experiential sources of meaning). Group meaning-centered psychotherapy has been proven to be more effective in reducing depression and hopelessness and improving quality of life in patients with advanced cancer, compared with supportive group psychotherapy.

Dignity therapy

Dignity therapy is a brief individual therapy designed to address existential distress in patients near the end of life. Dignity, a fundamental of one's psychological well-being, is considered to include themes of generativity and continuity of self, maintenance of pride and hope, role preservation, alleviation of concerns about being a burden to others, and the aftermath of his or her death. The dignity therapy counselor asks the patient questions related to the themes described earlier. The typical initial prompt is: "Tell me a little about your life history, particularly the parts that you either remember most or think were most important." The goal is to elicit the aspects of the patient's life that he or she considers meaningful or that he or she wants to be remembered for. The conversation between the patient and the therapist is tape-recorded, transcribed, edited, and passed on to the patient as a "generativity document," which can be shared with family.

CALM therapy

CALM therapy is a brief psychotherapy, currently being tested, which is designed to address specific problems that may be associated with psychological distress as well as psychological growth of patients with advanced cancer. It consists of four empirically derived domains of concern, namely, (a) symptom management and communication with health-care providers; (b) changes in self and relations with close others; (c) spirituality or sense of meaning and purpose; and (d) thinking of the future, hope, and mortality.

Systemic psychotherapies

Couple therapy. The needs, goals, and coping responses of patients and their partners are highly correlated and reciprocally interdependent. Couple therapy aims to enhance relationships and to protect patients and their partners against relational distress. It has been widely studied among breast cancer and prostate cancer populations.

Family therapy. Poor family function is associated with higher relapse rates of depression and the development of complicated grief. Family therapy, which aims to optimize family functioning through promotion of effective communication, enhanced cohesion, and adaptive resolution of conflict, was shown to reduce depression and support mourning after family loss due to cancer among low-functioning families.

Professional Issues and Service Implementation

Recording and Communicating

As described earlier, *depression* is a term whose meaning can range from usual sadness to clinical diagnosis of major depressive disorder. When a clinician uses the term *depression*, we must clarify what the term refers to clinically.

Severe Depression's Impact on Mental Capacity

Patients with severe depression are at elevated risk of suicide. If a patient is suspected to be at urgent risk of suicide, intensive psychiatric care, including one-to-one inpatient companionship on the oncology ward for safety or admission to a psychiatric ward, is indicated. In many countries, involuntary admission is permitted for patients who are at immediate risk of suicide. Clinicians are responsible for informing their caregivers of its risk, as well as referring such patients to an appropriate mental health care specialist. (See chapter 4 for more details on suicide risk management.)

Common Ethical Dilemmas

Depression is a large contributor to the wish for hastened death (e.g., thorough suicide, physician-assisted suicide, euthanasia, or rejection of proper treatment). Clinicians should be cautious about the presence of depression and its influence on patients with such requests. It is not always easy to discriminate clinical depression from a patient's natural response to tough physical conditions. The rule of thumb is to prioritize the diagnosis of depression in order not to miss the chance of recovery that can be attained.

Policies

Because of the high prevalence and remarkable impact of depression on patients' quality of life, some societies mandate routine screening of psychological distress (mainly targeting depression) in oncology practice. For example, the American College of Surgeons Commission on Cancer mandated implementation of a systematic protocol for distress screening and referral as a condition for cancer center accreditation starting in 2015. In Japan, provision of distress screening is required in order to be certified as a registered cancer center.

Teams and Supervision

Detection and management of depression may be best done by collaboration between front-line medical providers (e.g., primary care physicians or oncologists) and a trained "care manager" (e.g., trained nurses) who work under the supervision of consultant psychiatrists. A typical picture of this ostensible "collaborative care model" administering a self-report screening questionnaire for depression (e.g., HADS or PHQ-9) to all the patients in a clinic. If a patient reports high emotional distress, he or she receives a face-to-face or telephone diagnostic interview for depression by trained staff. If the patient is diagnosed with depression, he or she is provided with psychoeducation for depression and brief psychotherapy (usually brief CBT such as problem-solving therapy), in addition to practical advice on managing life with cancer and psychological distress. When clinically relevant, a report is generated for the patient's primary care provider. Also, a suggestion for use of psychotropics is provided by the care managers under the supervision of psychiatrists.

References

1. Mitchell AJ, Chan M, Bhatti H, et al. Prevalence of depression, anxiety, and adjustment disorder in oncological, haematological, and palliative-care settings: a meta-analysis of 94 interview-based studies. *Lancet Oncol.* 2011 Feb;12(2):160–174.

2. Fujisawa D, Inoguchi H, Shimoda H, et al. Impact of depression on health utility value in cancer patients. *Psychooncology* 2015;25(5):491–495. doi:10.1002/pon.3945

3. Pirl WF, Greer JA, Traeger L, et al. Depression and survival in metastatic non–small-cell lung cancer: effects of early palliative care. *J Clin Oncol.* 2012;30(12):1310–1315.

4. Warnke I, Nordt C, Kawohl W, Moock J, Rössler W. Age- and gender-specific mortality risk profiles for depressive outpatients with major chronic medical diseases. *J Affect Disord.* 2016;193:295–304. doi:10.1016/j.jad.2016.01.006

5. Mausbach BT, Schwab RB, Irwin SA. Depression as a predictor of adherence to adjuvant endocrine therapy (AET) in women with breast cancer: a systematic review and meta-analysis. *Breast Cancer Res Treat.* 2015;152(2):239–246. doi:10.1007/s10549-015-3471-7

6. Oliveira Miranda D, Soares de Lima TA, Ribeiro Azevedo L, Feres O, Ribeiro da Rocha JJ, Pereira-da-Silva G. Proinflammatory cytokines correlate with depression and anxiety in colorectal cancer patients. *Biomed Res Int.* 2014;739650. doi:10.1155/2014/739650

7. International Psycho-Oncology Society. IPOS International Standard of Quality Cancer Care. http://www.ipos-society.org/about-ipos/ipos-standard-of-quality-cancer-care/. Accessed May 31, 2016.

8. Andersen BL, DeRubeis RJ, Berman BS, Gruman J, Champion VL, Massie MJ, Holland JC, Partridge AH, Bak K, Somerfield MR, Rowland JH; American Society of Clinical Oncology. Screening, assessment, and care of anxiety and depressive symptoms in adults with cancer: an American Society of Clinical Oncology guideline adaptation. *J Clin Oncol.* 2014 May 20;32(15):1605–1619. doi:10.1200/JCO.2013.52.4611

9. Fujimori M, Shirai Y, Asai M, Kubota K, Katsumata N, Uchitomi Y. Effect of communication skills training program for oncologists based on patient preferences for communication when receiving bad news: a randomized controlled trial. *J Clin Oncol.* 2014;32(20):2166–2172. doi:10.1200/JCO.2013.51.2756.

10. Temel JS, Greer JA, Muzikansky A, et al. Early palliative care for patients with metastatic non-small-cell lung cancer. *N Engl J Med*. 2010;363(8):733–742. doi:10.1056/NEJMoa1000678

Further Reading

Akechi T, Ietsugu T, Sukigara M, et al. Symptom indicator of severity of depression in cancer patients: a comparison of the DSM-IV criteria with alternative diagnostic criteria. *Gen Hosp Psychiatry*. 2009;31(3):225–232.

This article shows the impact of diagnostic criteria upon the diagnosis of depressive disorders.

Akechi T, Okuyama T, Onishi J, Morita T, Furukawa TA. Psychotherapy for depression among incurable cancer patients. *Cochrane Database Syst Rev*. 2008 Apr. 16;(2):CD005537.

This is the only systematic review on psychotherapy for depression targeting incurable cancer patients.

Faller H, Schuler M, Richard M, Heckl U, Weis J, Kuffner R. Effects of psycho-oncologic interventions on emotional distress and quality of life in adult patients with cancer: systematic review and meta-analysis. *J Clin Oncol*. 2013;31:782–793.

This article reviews the effectiveness of psychosocial interventions for adult cancer patients.

Jacobsen PB, Jim HS. Psychosocial interventions for anxiety and depression in adult cancer patients: achievements and challenges. *CA-Cancer J Clin*. 2008;58(4):214–230.

This is a review of systematic reviews on psychosocial interventions for adult cancer patients.

Li M, Fitzgerald P, Rodin G. Evidence-based treatment of depression in patients with cancer. *J Clin Oncol*. 2012;30:1187–1196.

This article provides an evidence base for the selection of treatments for depression.

Luebbert K, Dahme B, Hasenbring M. The effectiveness of relaxation training in reducing treatment-related symptoms and improving emotional adjustment in acute non-surgical cancer treatment: a meta-analytical review. *Psychooncology*, 2001;10(6):490–502.

This article is a comprehensive review of relaxation for cancer patients.

Sharpe M, Walker J, Holm Hansen C, et al. Integrated collaborative care for comorbid major depression in patients with cancer (SMaRT Oncology-2): a multicentre randomised controlled effectiveness trial. *Lancet*. 2014;384(9948):1099–1108. doi:10.1016/S0140-6736(14)61231-9

This article describes the benefit of an integrated multidisciplinary model of care provision.

Wakefield CE, Butow PN, Aaronson NA, et al. Patient-reported depression measures in cancer: a meta-review. *Lancet Psychiatry*. 2015;2(7):635–647. doi:10.1016/S2215-0366(15)00168-6

This article will help guide readers in their selection of measures of clinical depression.

Chapter Quiz

1. Which conditions can mimic major depression in cancer patients?
   A. Medication-induced behavioral changes
   B. Physical symptom burden
   C. Hypoactive delirium
   D. All of the above

2. Which of the following symptoms indicate depression in cancer patients?
   A. Sleeplessness
   B. Diminished positive emotional reactions (e.g., no response to good news)
   C. Refusing medical care
   D. All of the above

3. Choose the correct description of *psychotropics*.
   A. Abrupt stopping of selective serotonin reuptake inhibitors (SSRI) or serotonin-norepinephrine reuptake inhibitors (SNRI) can cause withdrawal syndrome.
   B. Mirtazapine is an antidepressant that usually increases appetite.
   C. Anticholinergic effects often hamper use of tricyclic antidepressants (TCAs) in cancer patients.
   D. Benzodiazepine anxiolytics decrease wakefulness and can lead to delirium.
   E. All of the above

4. Which of the following sentences is correct? (choose one)
   A. Evidence is scarce on effectiveness of psychotherapy for cancer patients.
   B. All cancer patients are eligible for structured psychotherapy.
   C. Since depressed patients suffer from lack of energy, they are advised not to increase their activity level.
   D. Some of the psychotherapies can be provided by professionals who are not specialists in mental health if they receive a certain amount of training.

Chapter 3

Diagnosis and Treatment of Demoralization

David W. Kissane

Learning Objectives

After reading this chapter, the clinician will be able to
1. Recognize the contribution of meaning-based coping to adaptation and hope.
2. Discern the phenomenology of demoralization within patients' stories.
3. Differentiate diagnostic categories of mild, moderate, and severe demoralization, which may, in turn, lead to diagnoses of adjustment disorder with demoralization or major depression with demoralization.
4. Treat demoralization by appropriate selection of a range of cognitively informed, existentially oriented, and meaning-centered therapies to restore hope, morale, meaning, and purpose in life.

Background Evidence

Patients become demoralized when their morale drops as they cope with illness, its treatment, or any challenging predicament in which they find themselves. Lowered morale comes from some loss of hope about a situation that may be difficult to change, creating a sense of being stuck, trapped, or potentially helpless.[1] Persistence of this predicament can lead to growing pessimism and concern about the pointlessness of it all, leading the individual over time to potentially struggle to find meaning and purpose in the life that remains.[2] It can all seem too hard. There is risk of developing a sense of failure, which can lower self-esteem and self-worth and even create shame and doubt about the value of life. As all of this becomes intolerable, some patients develop suicidal thinking as they search for ways to escape this increasingly distressing state of mind.

Toward the end of the last century, a key revision of the conventional, theoretical model of coping, which saw the appraisal of any threat being responded to with *emotion-based* or *problem-based* coping, recognized the role of *meaning-based* coping as the third arm of each person's coping repertoire. Predicaments that bring an existential challenge about the value and worth of life are especially coped with via this meaning-based response.

It quickly becomes apparent that demoralization is a disorder of coping. Its conceptual advantage is that patients can readily understand this construct, acknowledge its presence, and welcome help to address it. Clinicians also understand this notion. As we shall see in this chapter, demoralization overlaps with both adjustment disorders and major depression. Time will tell whether the world chooses to formally recognize it as a separate diagnosis, the demoralization syndrome, or whether it will be used as a "specifier" to more accurately describe psychiatric diagnoses like adjustment disorder or major depression.[2] In this chapter, all three options will be illustrated. Demoralization is important diagnostically because it guides specific approaches to treatment that might not be selected if its presence were missed.

Demoralization is an ancient construct, described once in church literature as *acedia*—a tedious meaninglessness about life.[3] It was recognized in the psychosomatic era by G. Engel (1967) as the "given up–giving up" syndrome, by E. Gruenberg (1967) as the social breakdown of the chronically mentally ill, by J. Frank (1968) as the central issue to address in all effective psychotherapy, and by V. Frankl (1963) as one key expression of existential suffering[3,4] Demoralization can be precipitated by many aspects of illness but becomes most troublesome when the prognosis seems poor or the disease is progressive and nonresponsive to treatments, so that it truly becomes life-threatening.[4] Clinical states that can cause demoralization in patients include advanced cancer, incipient organ failure, progressive neurological disorders, substance dependence, chronic mental illness, poor symptom control, and the need for palliative care.

A recent systematic review found 25 studies of demoralization involving 4,545 patients in 10 countries.[2] Ten studies using the Demoralization Scale[5] identified a prevalence of clinically significant demoralization in the range of 13% to 18% of patients.[2] Moreover, this morbid state of mind is contagious in that it can be readily transmitted to family and friends, clinicians and care providers, lowering their morale as well. Demoralization thus becomes a major source of suffering.

Fang and colleagues demonstrated that demoralization is a more powerful mediator of suicidal ideation than depression.[6] Both depression and demoralization mediated the effects of psychological distress on suicidal ideation, with mediating effect sizes of 50% and 77%, respectively.[6] In a combined model exploring the mediating variables that contribute to the development of suicidal ideation, the overall mediating effect size was 75.4%, of which depression accounted for 18%, demoralization 25%, and depression × demoralization 31.8%.[6] Thus, a depressed patient with cancer who experiences demoralization will generate an increased effect on suicidal ideation by 50% to 75.4 % above the effect of depression alone.[6] These data point to the clinical importance of recognizing demoralization, where the loss of meaning and purpose proves to be the most powerful predictor of suicidal thinking.

Presenting Problems

Morale exists across a spectrum of mental states from high optimism at one end, through varied levels of low morale, to severe demoralization at the other end. Thus, looking dimensionally we can see (a) great positivity,

Table 3.1 Dimensional Nature of Demoralization

Nondemoralized Emotional States	Mild Demoralization	Moderate Demoralization	Severe Demoralization
Grief	Lack of confidence	Adjustment disorder	Despair
Fear	Disheartenment	Poor coping	Depression
Distress	Self-doubt	Self-failure	Suicidal

confidence, and determination (e.g., to win a sporting event); (b) mild loss of confidence, with disheartenment and self-doubt; (c) moderate demoralization with poor coping; and (d) severe demoralization associated with deep despair and risk of suicide. Recognizing this dimensional nature in the clinical setting, first mild cases of demoralization need to be differentiated from normal grief, fear, and distress that is proportional to the nature of the predicament (see Table 3.1).

Second, as the morbidity becomes more pathological and needs therapeutic assistance, moderate demoralization with some level of adjustment disorder emerges. At the far end of the spectrum, when severe demoralization becomes established, this mental state can be a harbinger of clinical depression or become comorbid with this psychiatric disorder.

Key Symptoms and Signs

Demoralization is a persisting mental state that arises as a result of a stressor event, often related to medical illness, with symptoms described in Box 3.1.

Box 3.1 Diagnostic Criteria for Demoralization

A. A poor sense of coping with an illness or predicament, occurring more days than not over the preceding two or more weeks
B. Feelings of low morale, reduced optimism, or nonspecific distress as a result of this struggle to cope
C. The poor coping and low morale are associated with **three (or more)** of the following:
  1. Hopelessness
  2. Helplessness or feeling stuck about being able to change the situation
  3. Pointlessness or loss of meaning
  4. Purposelessness
  5. Sense of failure or reduced self-worth as a person
  6. Doubts about the value of continued life
  7. Desire for hastened death
  8. Suicidal thoughts or plans
D. The poor coping or low morale cause clinically significant distress or impairment in social, occupational, or other important areas of functioning
E. The disturbance is not better explained by another mental or medical disorder

Table 3.2 Sociodemographic Factors Increasing Vulnerability for Demoralization

Predisposing/Perpetuating Factors	Protective Factors
Single, separated, divorced, widowed	Married or partnered
Living alone	Living with partner, family, friends
Reduced social support	Well supported
Unemployed	Employed
Low income/poverty	Financial security
Low self-esteem	Robust sense of self
Attachment insecurity	Secure attachments
Spiritual doubt	Spirituality or religious beliefs

Risk Factors

The risk factors that signify vulnerability to develop demoralization can be divided into (a) sociodemographic, (b) physical illness, (c) psychological and mental illness, and (d) treatment-related factors.[2] These need to be discerned through a comprehensive patient history.

Sociodemographic factors

These can predispose a person to or perpetuate demoralization or alternatively reflect resilience that will protect against its development as listed in Table 3.2.

Sociodemographic factors that are less clear-cut in predisposing to demoralization include age, gender, and education. However, high demoralization may be more prominent in women than men, in the less educated than the more educated, and in younger patients than elderly patients.[2]

Physical disease factors

These can also precipitate the acute onset of a demoralized state as described in Table 3.3.

Table 3.3 Physical Disease Factors Affecting Vulnerability for Demoralization

Predisposing/Precipitating/Perpetuating Factors	Protective Factors
Site of cancer (e.g., head and neck, brain)	Curable cancers
Progressive disease with poor prognosis	Good prognosis cancer
Debilitating diseases (e.g., motor neurone disease)	Well-controlled disease or cancer

Poor symptom control
  Difficult pain
  Breathing problems
  Chronic fatigue
  Cognitive problems
  Mobility constraints
	Good quality of life
	  Optimal symptom control

Table 3.4 Psychological Factors Affecting Vulnerability for Demoralization

Predisposing/Precipitating/Perpetuating Factors	Protective Factors
Chronic distress/dysthymia	Hopefulness, purpose in life
Clinical depression	Happiness, joy
Clinical anxiety	Peace and calm, safety
Suicidality	Will to live, interest in life
Somatization	Good quality of life
Chronic mental illness with treatment resistance, functional decline, or social isolation	Robust inner life

No significant associations have been found between demoralization and the time since diagnosis, stage of disease, or range of treatments used to manage the illness.[2] In contrast with the range of treatments, specific treatment complications precipitating demoralization are considered in Table 3.5.

Psychological or mental illness factors
A past history of limited coping or clinical depression can reflect a personal vulnerability when a stressor of sufficient intensity presents itself, as shown in Table 3.4.

Treatment-related factors
Some treatments will cause disfigurement with resultant potential for stigma and shame, interference with relationships, and altered quality of life. Others will cause significant side effects, resulting in increased burden of symptomatology and a consequential challenge to coping, as shown in Table 3.5.

While any one or a combination of vulnerability factors has the potential to increase the risk of demoralization, the cumulative build-up of several factors increases the likelihood of reduced coping, no matter how resilient the individual first appeared.[2,4]

How to make a diagnosis and assess need. A comprehensive history and mental state examination is required in a clinical interview. As this unfolds, the clinician attends to both the patient's sense of coping and his

Table 3.5 Treatment-Related Factors Increasing Vulnerability for Demoralization

Precipitating/Perpetuating Factors	Protective Factors
Amputations, stoma	Keyhole or robotic surgery
Surgical morbidity	Surgery complication free
Long-term or late effects of radiation	Complication-free radiotherapy
Adverse chemotherapy side effects	Well-tolerated chemotherapy
Chronic pain syndromes	Good quality of life
Chemotherapy resistance	Good cancer or disease control

or her morale when speaking about it. *Take note of the diagnostic criteria for demoralization as shown in Box 3.1, p. 45.* The following case studies will illustrate typical patient histories and highlight the differences between demoralization, clinical depression, and the more severe situation of major depression with melancholia.

Factors that may contribute to misdiagnosis. A clinician can miss the diagnosis of demoralization by not asking questions that explore the patient's morale and sense of coping. A focus on physical symptoms without asking psychosocial questions will miss the diagnosis in a patient who remains silent about his or her morale, possibly sensing the clinician's discomfort with his or her predicament.

Case Study

First we review a patient with an adjustment disorder with demoralization. In this vignette, watch for relevant phenomenology that would point to this diagnosis.

Adjustment Disorder with Demoralization

Alice is a 50-year old, divorced school teacher and mother of two who has been receiving chemotherapy treatment for advanced lung cancer, with bony and liver secondaries. Two weeks ago, Alice received news of disease progression on CT imaging. She had been on fourth line chemotherapy in the hope of containing her cancer's spread. Her oncologist mentioned that they were running out of options, which left Alice sitting silently, thinking that her days were now numbered. She shrugged her shoulders and left the oncologist's room with tears in her eyes but resolute that she would remain composed.

Today, Alice is visiting her general practitioner to get a refill of her bronchodilator medication. She has a long face and looks disheartened. When asked how her cancer treatment was going, Alice says that there doesn't seem to be much point to chemotherapy anymore. It has not stopped the growth of her cancer. Alice adds that life has not been the same since she stopped working. She misses seeing her friends. She had been preoccupied with her children's secondary school in years gone by, but since they had completed college and lived independently, she saw much less of them. They were busy with their jobs, partners, and all the activities that kept them occupied.

The doctor asks Alice how she is feeling. "My mood's okay, Doctor," she says. "I'm good when my head is in a good book or I'm watching a favorite movie. Just not sure where my life is going. The world is leaving me behind. There does not seem to be much to get up for these days. I wondered if I killed myself would anyone miss me, but I guess it would make my family sad." The doctor asks Alice directly if she feels depressed. "No, Doctor, I've still got my sense of humor. I'm eating, sleeping well, I enjoy a movie on TV. There just doesn't seem to be much point to life since I stopped work. I find myself thinking, 'Why bother?' I guess it is hard to keep my spirits up when I know the oncology doctors can't do much more to help me."

The doctor asks Alice if she'd like more help. "Nah, Doc. I'll be okay. It's just that when the doctors don't hold much hope for you, it impacts your morale. The tennis final is on this afternoon. Doctor, who do you think will win the game?"

Key features in the patient named Alice

In this account, Alice reports lowered morale and reduced hope arising in the context of limited disease-containing treatment options for her advanced cancer. Alice denies feeling depressed and is not anhedonic. She tries to rally herself, with reference to sources of pleasure such as the tennis match, a book, or a movie, but she doubts the value of the future ("not sure where my life is going") in a life in which she is not working, and there is reduced meaning ("not much to get up for") and loss of purpose ("doesn't seem to be much point"). Alice fleetingly contemplates suicide but dismisses this because of the impact it might have on her children.

Here the stressor is the loss of chemotherapy control over her illness, with resultant distress and impaired functioning. Vulnerability factors include her young age, single status, reduced contact with her children, and not socializing with her friends. Acute grief would be a culturally normative response in many Western communities, but instead of sharing her grief, Alice focuses on the loss of meaning, purpose, and hope for a future with sustained value in life. Alice cannot anticipate a worthwhile future. The clinical judgement here is that Alice's response is maladaptive; her demoralization is a poor coping response, as she appears to be getting stuck in this state of mind, without an ability to hope for a reasonable quality of life while she takes one day at a time. The development of courage and the capacity to live in the present moment are challenges for many people.

Alice would not meet diagnostic criteria for a major depressive episode (a clinical depression), nor does she display features of overt anxiety as might be found in a person with generalized anxiety disorder. She does, however, have an adjustment disorder, whose specifier would be most aptly termed "with demoralization." Alternative specifiers such as "with depressed mood," "with anxious mood," or "with mixed features" do not capture her mental state accurately. The value of the diagnosis of adjustment disorder with demoralization is that this guides a clinician to psychotherapy that specifically addresses her demoralization. We will deal with the treatment of demoralization later in this chapter.

First let us consider a different patient where the features of a major depression have developed and yet demoralization is comorbidly present. Watch for the phenomenology that would point to the diagnosis of major depressive disorder with demoralization.

Case Study

Major Depression with Demoralization

George is a 52-year-old man who, for 15 months, has been battling pancreatic cancer that was inoperable at diagnosis because of its size and involvement of the mesenteric artery. After initial chemo-radiation therapy, George learned that secondary spread to the liver had occurred. Despite further treatment with two regimens of chemotherapy, his oncologist reported that the cancer had progressed again on imaging and was aggressive in nature. George feels hopeless and helpless, fearing that his days are numbered and wondering what is the point of it all.

George is married with two daughters and has worked as an accountant. His wife is a nurse and often accompanies him on his medical visits. She worries that George has become depressed, and indeed George reports a persisting low mood over the past month, ever since he learned of his last imaging result. He finds himself thinking often about his death, losing his sense of joy, ruminating in the middle of the night, losing his appetite and 4 kg of weight, and feeling fatigued, with poor concentration, reduced interest in the news and TV, low energy, no libido, and little motivation to do things differently.

George says he feels stuck, trapped with a disease that will kill him, with a growing sense that his doctors are going through the motions but not able to really help him. Since he stopped work a couple of months back, his life has lost meaning and he has little to get up for in the morning. He reports despair, commenting that all of this treatment seems a waste of time, that perhaps he'd be better off "being put down" as there is no hope for a better future. When at his lowest, he has thought of swallowing all of his pills, but he hasn't acted for fear of upsetting his wife and family. He copes by spending more time in bed, preferring to pull the covers over his head and quietly wait for whatever must happen.

George looks a little disheveled, appearing sad with a flat affect, and talking about the pointlessness of it all. He has no hope for a better future and wonders if death isn't the inescapable answer.

Key features in the patient named George

George has the classical features for a major depressive episode, with persisting depressed mood over a four-week period, reduced interest and anhedonia, accompanied by fatigue, anorexia, weight loss, insomnia, poor concentration, and suicidal thoughts. What is noteworthy about his depression is the hopelessness and helplessness, meaninglessness, and purposelessness that dominates his thinking and leads him to suicidal thinking. He is stuck in this mindset and uses withdrawal and avoidant coping, and his suffering becomes profound as a result. In addition to treatment with antidepressants, psychotherapy for his demoralization will prove worthwhile.

Demoralization versus Melancholia

A specifier such as "melancholia" can be used with a diagnosis of major depression to identify a more serious form of depression. This can be differentiated from demoralization. The features of melancholia include

A. Either (a) loss of pleasure in almost all activities or (b) loss of reactivity to usually pleasurable activities

B. Plus three or more of the following:
  1. Distinct mood quality of profound moroseness, emptiness, despondence, or despair
  2. Diurnal variation—depression is worse in the morning
  3. Early morning awakening
  4. Marked psychomotor retardation or agitation
  5. Very significant anorexia or weight loss
  6. Excessive guilt

Patients with an agitated depression can wring their hands, pace about, and appear agitated, while the patient with slow thinking and reduced movement stands out with these features of psychomotor retardation. The diurnal patterns reflect biological changes tied to circadian rhythm. Although the melancholic patient has profound features of depression with distinct phenomenology, they differ in key ways from demoralization.

Although the demoralized can exhibit a deep despair, the cognitions that accompany this focus on hopelessness, helplessness, worthlessness, meaningless, and loss of purpose. The demoralized's rumination about the loss of anticipatory pleasure in the future is noteworthy. The biological aspects of melancholia, where the patient's face is nonreactive, with the passive nonexpressiveness found in psychomotor retardation, are not present. Both sets of phenomena can convey a sense of accompanying subjective incompetence, feeling stuck in their predicament, but the demoralized person contemplates suicide as the solution, while the melancholic has almost lost the drive to plan this. The melancholic's more natural way forward is nihilistic thinking, where the body is perceived to be dead already.

These differences are subtle. The clinician must strive to understand the mindset of each person, to listen thoughtfully to his or her ideas, and to comprehend his or her cognitions about their life. We illustrate with a clinical vignette of a patient with a major depression with melancholia.

Case Study

Major Depression with Melancholia

Stan is a 60-year-old man with progressive gastric cancer, with liver and lung secondaries failing to be controlled now by his fifth regimen of chemotherapy. Stan has felt morose and empty over the past month, all the pleasure appearing to go from his life. He feels depressed when he wakes early in the morning, around 4 AM, feels slowed down with no energy, can't make decisions, has no appetite, has had a profound weight loss of 30 kg, and feels guilty that he cannot find any happiness in his days.

Stan had been an engineer, who had always been a stellar provider. There had not been anything remarkable in his past history until this cancer came along. Stan had always been interested in politics and was generally a friendly, intelligent, and warm character. His wife described him as "a good man and a man of faith."
Stan is accompanied by an anxious wife, who helps him walk into your consulting room. He looks despondent and stares ahead when the doctor asks him questions. His responses are slow in coming, as if he is searching for what to say. He laments that he shouldn't feel so down and is upsetting his family too much. There is no responsiveness when the doctor attempts to brighten the situation. What has happened is a mystery to him. He denies any suicidal thinking, commenting that he feels bewildered about it all.

Key features in the patient named Stan
A patient with melancholia, like Stan, has a distinct flavor to his phenomenology that is quite different from the demoralized. The psychomotor slowing,

diurnal pattern and distinct facies leap out at the clinician who meets Stan. Although the oncologist might be struck by cancer cachexia, the psychiatrist looks beyond this to the nature and quality of mental processes. An inclusive approach to considering cancer-related symptomatology alongside vegetative symptoms of depression ensures that the melancholia is not missed, as it requires the treatment of the clinical depression in quite specific ways.

Investigations for Key Differential Diagnoses

The workup, outlined in chapter 2 (differential diagnosis for clinical depression) to rule out key physical conditions, medication effects, organic brain disorders, and other severe psychiatric disorders applies here. While less important for adjustment disorder with demoralization, once the more severe demoralization that can be found accompanying major depression or melancholia occurs, this careful medical workup is worthwhile.

Assessment of the severity of demoralization can be achieved through the use of the Demoralization Scale (see Appendix 2). If measured at baseline, follow-up measurement as psychotherapeutic treatment of the demoralization occurs allows this monitoring to demonstrate clinical improvement over time. The original pencil-and-paper measure of demoralization, the 24-item, five-factor Demoralization Scale (DS), was validated in 2004.[5] This was translated into several languages, and its factor structure was found to vary between cultures.[2] A refinement and revalidation was undertaken into a shorter, 16-item, two-factor Demoralization Scale-II (DS-II), with stronger psychometric properties. For the DS-II, the response format of the DS was collapsed by Rasch analysis (item response theory modelling) into a 3-point format.[7] Internal consistency of the total DS-II was Cronbach's $\alpha = 0.89$, with the eight-item Meaning and Purpose subscale at Cronbach's $\alpha = 0.84$ and the eight-item Distress and Coping Ability subscale at Cronbach's $\alpha = 0.82$.[7] Test–retest reliability in a stable clinical setting showed an intraclass correlation coefficient $= 0.80$.

Convergent validity of the DS-II was strong with measures of psychological distress, existential well-being, quality of life, and attitudes toward end-of-life, including will to live and desire to die.[8] Discriminant validity was evident in differentiating patients with different Karnofsky functional performance levels and high versus low symptom scores on the Memorial Symptom Assessment Scale.[8] At severe levels of demoralization, comorbidity with depression occurs, while moderate levels of demoralization appear independent of clinical depression.[8]

Items of the DS-II are reproduced for clinical use in Appendix 2 (see page 110). Clinical studies in advanced cancer have found median levels of 6 on the DS-II,[7] with a threshold of ≥ 8 indicative of clinical concern. A minimal clinically meaningful difference was found to be 2 points, while an improvement of >4 points has been found with effective symptom management in palliative care populations.[8]

Clinical Management

Next we consider mild, moderate, and severe forms of demoralization in turn.

Figure 3.1 lays out an algorithm indicating the broad management strategies employed to help the demoralized. Note that the severity of demoralization is assessed alongside risk or vulnerability factors, which may be also be worthwhile therapeutic targets.

Mild Demoralization—Supportive Psychotherapy

Mild demoralization, which can fluctuate and be short-lived, may be assuaged by empathic listening and supportive psychotherapy, where the key components of this intervention are

- Empathic acknowledgement of the patient's plight (e.g. "You are in a terribly difficult situation").

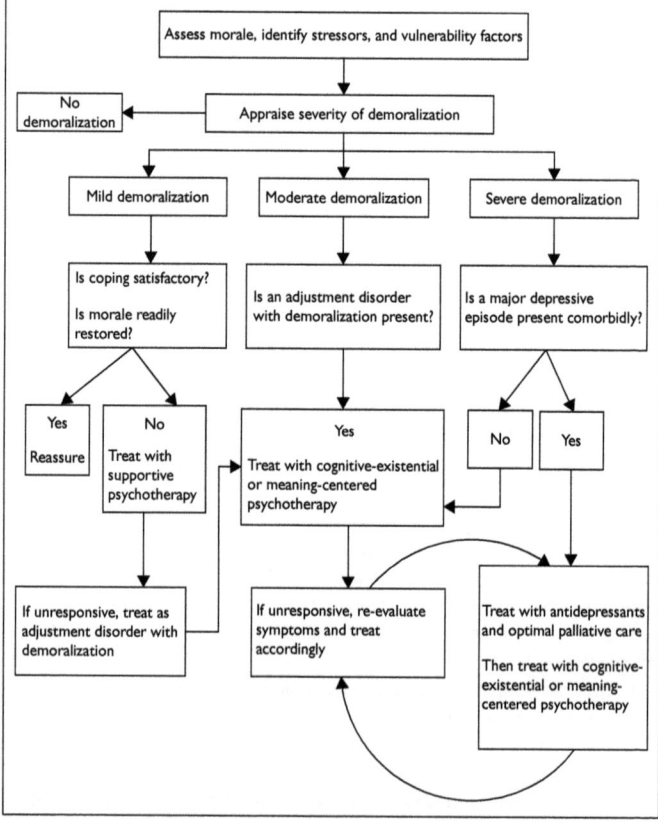

Figure 3.1. Overall guide to the management of demoralization.

- Normalization of grief and distress (e.g. "Your tears are both appropriate and normal. ... we call this grief").
- Affirmation of the person's strengths and sources of resilience (e.g. "You strike me as a determined person, who has wisely known when to share your grief with your loved ones and gained from their support").
- Encouragement to adapt with courage and sustain focus on living in the moment (e.g., "I admire your courage as a key strength of your coping. You are setting goals for each day. Keep striving to live in the moment").

Brief psychotherapy at the bedside or in the consultation room employs questions about existential concerns that impact the patient's morale.[9] The clinician monitors this on a regular basis, clarifying understanding of the illness and the goals of treatment, correcting any misunderstanding of the prognosis, and identifying sources of hope for the future.

Examination of spirituality, religious beliefs, or philosophy of life can be helpful if the patient has a belief system that might be a source of help or inspiration at this time. Is there hope for a life beyond this life? Some form of rebirth? Some form of continuity within family memories transmitted from one generation to the next? Can spiritual peace and consolation be used to buffer the disappointment that might arise from disease progression? Are there particular rituals within a religious tradition that might apply at this time?

This model of clinical responsiveness to mild demoralization does not seek to pathologize this state of mind but rather recognizes the role of the clinician's support as the means to assist the common and mild fluctuations in morale that occur naturally across the illness trajectory.

Moderate Demoralization—Combinations of Cognitive-Existential and Meaning-Centered Therapy

Cognitively oriented approaches

Cognitively oriented approaches recognize thinking distortions arising from pessimism, catastrophization, exaggeration, or selective focus on the negative. Exemplary questions include

- Is the clinical understanding of illness and prognosis realistic?
- Are there negative emotional consequences that arise from the patient's thinking that handicap his or her coping response?
- Can reframing of negative cognitions help restore morale?

(See brief outline of cognitive behavioral therapy techniques in Chapter 2.)

Existentially oriented approaches

Existentially oriented approaches invite the patient to acknowledge the finitude of life, the cost of anticipatory grief, and the burden of fear and worry about what might happen in the future versus the benefits that flow from a sustained focus on "living in the moment" and "keeping on living." The conclusion drawn from more than a century's worth of philosophical examination of the problem of mortality is that an orientation toward life with all its richness, engagement, and creativity is what is most important to our common human existence. Exemplary questions include

- What is the burden of your preoccupation with your grief?
- Does this worry about what might happen help you?

- What is most important in your life right now?
- What does it mean to you when people suggest that we all "live in the moment"?

Both Yalom's classic text *Existential Psychotherapy* and Spiegel and Classen's supportive-expressive group therapy model employ existentially oriented therapies (see Further Reading).

Note that cognitively and existentially oriented therapies can be readily combined in clinical practice.[10]

Meaning-centered therapy

This therapy recognizes the centrality of the quest for meaning in human life and invites the patient to consider the many and varied sources of meaning that exist in his or her life.[11] A narrative therapy approach to understanding the patient's life can make use of an inventory of meaning-centered questions (see Box 3.2) to guide the patient's reflection in this direction. This inventory of meaning-centered questions presents an overall catalogue of themes from which a clinician can select and tailor questions to suit the specific individual. In each case,

---

Box 3.2 Inventory of Meaning-Centered Questions

- Sources of fulfillment
  i. What accomplishments are you most proud of? Have you had a mission in your life?
  ii. What legacy will you leave? How do you want to be remembered?
  iii. Did you make a contribution through your profession or working life?
  iv. Did you make a contribution to your family, country or community?
  v. What were you like at the top of your game?
- Roles in life
  i. What is your role as a spouse or parent? Sibling? Grandparent? Friend?
  ii. How can you sustain engagement with roles that have mattered to you?
  iii. What tasks or deeds remain in your various roles within the family?
- Sources of creativity
  i. Do you have an appreciation of music? Art? Beauty? Humor?
  ii. Have you had passions, hobbies, obsessions through the years?
  iii. Are there letters you could write? Stories that you want to tell?
  iv. Who have been your major loves?
- Attitude or philosophy about life
  i. What have been your sources of motivation and commitment to life?
  ii. Has there been a set of values that you have lived by?
  iii. Is there anyone whose needs you would put ahead of your own?
  iv. Can you sustain an attitude toward keeping meaning alive in your life? Be determined to do this?
- Acceptance of self
  i. Are there limitations, regrets, or wrongs that warrant acceptance?

(continued)

> **Box 3.2 (Continued)**
>
> ii. Can a wholesomeness, worthiness, or "goodness that is sufficient" be recognized?
> iii. Is there a place for forgiveness?
> iv. Is there anything you want to finish, improve, or resolve?
> v. How do you learn to live "ill"? Disabled? Disfigured?
> vi. What best defines your character as a person?
>
> - Meaningful relationships
>   i. Who has mattered in your life? Who still matters?
>   ii. Are there any concerns for your family?
>   iii. What is the place of gratitude for all that you have shared?
> - Identity and impact of cancer
>   i. Do you hold on to your sense of worth and value as a person?
>   ii. Has the illness impacted in significant ways on who you are?
>   iii. Can you accept the changes in your body? Its frailty?
> - Deepening of generalized hope
>   i. Dare you hope for improved quality of life? Can you hope to learn to live "ill," perhaps less well but still with some quality?
>   ii. Dare you hope for rebirth? For passage to a continued spiritual existence? For God?
>   iii. Do you recognize an inner hope that transcends the ordinary particular hopes in life?
>   iv. Can you hope that your survivors benefit from knowing you?
> - Continuing responsibilities
>   i. What ongoing responsibilities are there that warrant your effort and commitment?
>   ii. What gifts can you leave?
>   iii. Who might profit from your affirmation?
>   iv. Can you help to prepare your loved ones for what lies ahead? What could you do to teach your grandchildren about being elderly and ill? About dying?
>   v. How will conversations about leaving, dying, and saying "goodbye" and "thank you" occur?
>   vi. Can you live life out to the fullest, until the very moment when it stops?

the question is intended to stimulate a reflective process; each response can evoke further curiosity and lead to considerable discussion. Models of therapy like CALM (Managing Cancer and Living Meaningfully),[12] meaning and purpose therapy,[13] and meaning-centered therapy/meaning-centered group therapy[11] build on this process across several sessions to develop each person's sense of meaning, will to live, and focus of priorities in his or her life.

Family-centered support

Demoralization has a contagious nature. When people who feel hopeless and trapped convey this emotionally to their relatives and friends, they in turn (especially when they fail to rally the morale of the patient) can feel hopeless and stuck as well. The clinician does well to remember the need to talk with the family, determine the level of their morale, and help them in turn with their coping.

A family meeting can be an essential component of care provision. This meeting can focus on the following goals:
- Review the stage of the illness, its status and prognosis.
- Review the goals of care, including the importance of hope.
- Check up on family communication, teamwork, and coping.
- Educate and support the family in their caregiving role.

Families are greatly helped by the provision of an opportunity to talk together about many of these issues and concerns, guided by the experience of the treating team. They need to be reminded that the patient, who is frail and ill, has often had some time to adjust to this level of bodily dysfunction, while the onlooker perceives this change as acute and horrible. Families need to have their needs considered and resources provided to them as appropriate.

A model of family-centered care can be employed in which families at risk because of some restriction in their open communication, ready teamwork and mutual support, or capacity to resolve their differences and conflicts are engaged during palliative care in a program of 6 to 10 family meetings over 12 to 18 months.[14] This has been shown in clinical trials to prevent complicated grief (e.g., prolonged grief disorder) through the relational support the family receives. (For resources, see Kissane and Bloch, and Kissane and Parnes in Further Reading).

Severe Demoralization

The following principles summarize the management of severe demoralization:

- **Active symptom management** of all aggravating symptoms—control pain, nausea, constipation, dyspnoea, insomnia, and depression; use antidepressants for anhedonic depression. Maintain continuity of care throughout.
- **Explore attitudes about hope and meaning** in life using narrative therapies that review the patient's life story (see the section on management of moderate demoralization for approaches to existential and meaning-centered psychotherapy).
- **Balance support for grief with promotion of hope and discussion of transitions** in life, so that acceptance of change is nurtured; the use of aspects of interpersonal therapy is apt here. Most role changes in life involve loss as well as opportunity.
- **Foster search for renewed purpose and role in life**, using aspects of interpersonal therapy and meaning-centered psychotherapy.
- **Promote supportive relationships and use of community volunteers**, especially for the lonely and isolated.
- **Use cognitive therapy** to reframe negative beliefs.
- **Conduct family meetings** to enhance family functioning and protect against the development of family demoralization.

- **Review goals of care** in multidisciplinary team meetings to ensure that the entire treatment team is engaged in this management plan.

Many of the questions and techniques described in the management of moderate demoralization (adjustment disorder with demoralization) apply as well to severe demoralization, including major depression with demoralization. *Using pharmacotherapy to better control symptoms and distress is necessary before a patient may be ready and psychologically available for psychotherapy.* Use of antidepressants, where the dose is appropriately titrated over time, in the setting of major depression is thus important. Wisdom and experience is needed to guide the timing of what to introduce when. Although a range of themes and potential issues are specified in lists in this chapter, the clinician must exercise judgement about the pace and selection of options in keeping with the patient's readiness to engage and respond to these issues.

Priorities Using Hypothetical Time Lines

A useful exercise to help either an individual patient or a couple prioritize and set goals for the future is to have them create a hypothetical list of their wishes and plans across short-term, mid-range and longer term time periods. The clinician can adjust the time periods proportional to the prognosis of the patient. Thus, for patients with an approximate prognosis of six months, invite them to create lists for 3-, 6-, and 12-month periods; for patients with a prognosis of one to two years, invite them to consider time lines of 6 to 12 months, 18 months, and 3 years. Each party is asked to draw up a personal list and then the individual or couple are invited to share their ideas and discuss the reasons behind each choice. While the focus of the exercise is on working toward agreement about their priorities for the future, the hypothetical time line exercise helps couples to talk about mortality and the uncertainty that people inevitably face.

Presence, Listening, and Accompaniment

Hospice and palliative care services have learned the importance of the clinician remaining committed and reviewing how the patient is doing and coping. At the heart of this is both building and sustaining a relationship with the patient and family. It is well recognized that some clinicians will avoid entering the room of a dying patient, with the clinician's withdrawal pointing to awkwardness and personal issues with mortality and death. The quality of patient care can suffer when clinicians have not worked through their personal issues about the finitude of life. Death anxiety is universal and as much a challenge to the clinician as to the patient and family.

Honest reflection about countertransference, avoidant behaviors, spirituality, and philosophy of life are vital for the clinician to exercise personal courage and identify what is needed to accompany the dying, to sit by the patient's bed, and to honor the dignity of the person the clinician has come to know and value as a fellow human being.

Recognition of our common humanity is the cornerstone to compassionate and competent clinical care that can ameliorate demoralization and sustain our continued living until we die.

Professional Issues and Service Implementation

Challenges for multidisciplinary teams caring for patients with advanced cancer are similar to those for families and include

- Watching bodily decay and frailty with horror and dismay.
- Distress at poor symptom control.
- Sense of helplessness that they cannot fix all that is happening.
- Strain of care provision and feeling burdened.
- Undeclared conflict and tension between viewpoints.

Ethical dilemmas arise for teams when demoralized patients or families ask for help with physician-assisted suicide. See chapter 2 for discussion of euthanasia and depression and chapter 4 for discussion of the suicidal patient.

References

1. Kissane DW. Demoralization—A life-preserving diagnosis to make in the severely medically ill. *J Pall Care.* 2014;30(4):255–258.
2. Robinson S, Kissane DW, Brooker J, Burney S. A systematic review of the demoralization syndrome in individuals with progressive disease and cancer: a decade of research. *J Pain Symp Manage.* 2015;49(3):595–610. doi:10.1016/j.jpainsymman.2014.07.008
3. Kissane DW, Clarke DM, Street AF. Demoralization syndrome—a relevant psychiatric diagnosis for palliative care. *J Pall Care.* 2001;17:12–21.
4. Robinson S, Kissane DW, Brooker J, Burnie S. A review of the construct of demoralization: history, definitions and future. *Am J Hosp Pall Med.* 2016;33(1):93–101. doi:10.1177/1049909114553461
5. Kissane DW, Wein S, Love A, Lee XQ, Kee PL, Clarke DM. The Demoralization Scale: a preliminary report of its development and preliminary validation. *J Pall Care.* 2004;20(4):269–276.
6. Fang CK, Chang MC, Chen PJ, et al. A correlational study of suicidal ideation with psychological distress, depression, and demoralization in patients with cancer. *Support Care Cancer.* 2014;22(12):3165–3174. doi:10.1007/s00520-014-2290-4
7. Robinson S, Kissane DW, Brooker J, et al. Refinement and revalidation of the Demoralization Scale: The DS-II—internal validity. *Cancer.* 2016;122(14):2251–2259.
8. Robinson S, Kissane DW, Brooker J, et al. Refinement and revalidation of the Demoralization Scale: DS-II—external validity. *Cancer.* 2016;122(14):2260–2667.
9. Griffith JL, Gaby L. Brief psychotherapy at the bedside: countering demoralization from medical illness. *Psychosomatics.* 2005;46(2):109–116. doi:http://dx.doi.org/10.1176/appi.psy.46.2.109

10. Kissane DW, Miach P, Bloch S, Seddon A, Smith GC. Cognitive-existential group therapy for patients with primary breast cancer. *Psychooncology*. 1997; 6:25–33.
11. Breitbart W, Rosenfeld B, Pessin H, Applebaum A, Kulikowski J, Lichtenthal WG. Meaning-centered group psychotherapy: an effective intervention for improving psychological well-being in patients with advanced cancer. *J Clin Oncol*. 2015;33(7):749–754. doi:10.1200/JCO.2014.57.2198
12. Lo C, Hales S, Jung J, et al. Managing Cancer And Living Meaningfully (CALM): phase 2 trial of a brief individual psychotherapy for patients with advanced cancer. *Palliat Med*. 2014;28(3):234–242. doi:10.1177/0269216313507757
13. Lethborg C, Schofield P, Kissane DW. The advanced cancer patient experience of undertaking meaning and purpose (MaP) therapy. *Palliat Support Care*. 2012;10(3):177–188. doi:10.1017/S147895151100085X
14. Kissane DW, Zaider TI, Li Y, et al. Randomized controlled trial of family therapy in advanced cancer. *J Clin Oncol*. 2016;34(16):1921–1927.

Further Reading

Breitbart WS, Poppito S. *Individual Meaning-Centered Therapy for Patients with Advanced Cancer: A Treatment Manual*. New York: Oxford University Press; 2014.

Manual to guide this psychoeducational approach to fostering meaning.

Frank JD, Frank JB. *Persuasion and Healing: A Comparative Study of Psychotherapy*. 3rd ed. Baltimore: Johns Hopkins University Press; 1991.

Classic book about the importance of restoring hope and morale in all psychotherapy.

Kissane DW, Bloch S. *Family-Focused Grief Therapy*. Chichester, UK: Open University Press; 2002.

Model of family-centered care that supports the family and fosters their engagement with the patient for as long as possible.

Kissane DW, Parnes F. *Bereavement Care for Families*. New York: Routledge; 2014.

Further elaboration of family-centered care during palliative care and extended into bereavement.

Spiegel D, Classen C. *Group Therapy for Cancer Patients: A Research-Based Handbook of Psychosocial Care*. New York: Basic Books; 2000.

Classic account of supportive-expressive therapy as an existentially and meaning-centered approach.

Watson M, Kissane DW. *Handbook of Psychotherapy in Cancer Care*. London: Wiley; 2010.

International Psycho Oncology Society–endorsed textbook about the delivery of models of psychotherapy in cancer care.

Yalom ID. *Existential Psychotherapy*. London: Basic Books; 1980.

The most accessible and classic account of existential psychotherapy.

Chapter Quiz

Read the following clinical vignette and select the best answers from the choices that follow.

Tony is a 55-year-old lawyer, married with two adolescent children, who has been receiving treatment for two years for advanced melanoma, which has spread to his liver and brain. An occipital cerebral metastasis was resected, followed by stereotactic radiation. For 10 months, Tony responded to treatment with Ipilimumab, a monoclonal antibody that activates T-cells. Molecular diagnostics on his melanoma had confirmed a BRAF mutation, making him suitable to then go on to treatment with the programmed death (PD-1) receptor antagonist, Nivolumab. Again, there was disease containment for some months before imaging showed regrowth of his liver secondaries, this time more substantially. Tony's oncologist has been hinting that his treatment options are running out. This causes Tony dismay, and he speaks of feeling trapped unfairly by this illness while still a young man. He still enjoys his work, but he wonders what the point is going forward. He tells his oncologist that life appears futile now. He asks if he should be put down like a dog. His oncologist is perturbed and mystified about how best to help Tony.

1. What is the most useful diagnosis for this patient? (choose one)
   A. Normal grief reaction or normal situational reaction
   B. Adjustment disorder
   C. Adjustment disorder with anxiety
   D. Adjustment disorder with depressed mood
   E. Adjustment disorder with demoralization
   F. Major depressive disorder
   G. Major depressive disorder with melancholia
   H. Major depressive disorder with demoralization

2. What is the best treatment for this patient? (choose one)
   A. Reassurance
   B. Supportive counseling or supportive psychotherapy
   C. Meaning-centered therapy or existential psychotherapy
   D. Cognitive-behavioral therapy
   E. Antidepressant medication with cognitive-behavioral therapy
   F. Antidepressant medication with meaning-centered therapy or existential psychotherapy
   G. Antidepressant medication with supportive counseling
   H. Antianxiety medication

# Chapter 4

Recognizing and Managing Suicide Risk

Maggie Watson and Luigi Grassi

Learning Objectives

After reading this chapter, the clinician will be able to
1. Critically appraise the background evidence on suicide rates and risk factors.
2. Evaluate presenting problems involving suicide risk.
3. Undertake investigations key to evaluating the differential diagnosis.
4. Apply clinical management options.
5. Recognize professional issues (i.e., policymaking and service implementation, including legal and clinical responsibilities in managing suicide and suicide risk).

Background Evidence

Suicide Rates

The number of completed suicides among cancer patients is between 1.5 to 2 times greater than the general population,[1,2] with rates being greater among cancer patients than those with other medical conditions.[3] Suicidal ideation/thoughts are common in cancer patients with rates between 7% to 40%.[4–7]

Suicide Risk Factors

Common risk factors include male gender, social disruption/isolation (e.g., through separation, divorce, or widowhood), older age, current/past history of psychiatric disorders, and substance abuse. The most important factor is represented by a psychiatric diagnosis, particularly clinical depression, demoralization, and substance abuse. More specifically, if a psychiatric disorder is characterized by suicidal ideation with elevated intentionality, marked anxiety and agitation, and poor impulse control, the risk of suicide dramatically increases. Patients suffering from mood disorder, especially unipolar major depression or bipolar disorders, schizophrenia, and substance abuse disorders, are at increased risk of suicide. Patients with personality disorders and posttraumatic stress disorders can also be at higher risk of suicide. *Patients in these mental health categories who develop cancer should be monitored with extreme care and attention.*

Cancer-Related Risk Factors

Apart from psychiatric disorders, type of cancer and cancer-related conditions have a role in increasing risk of suicide ideation and completed suicide. The highest rates have been recorded in patients with lung, stomach, and head and neck cancers.[1,8] In a study of stomach-cancer survivors, findings indicated a high rate of suicide ideation (about 35%) that was significantly associated with psychological symptoms (e.g., emotional functioning), as well as physical functioning and cancer-related symptoms (e.g., fatigue, nausea/vomiting, dyspnoea, and appetite loss).[9] The first year after cancer diagnosis is considered a period of higher risk.[10] An advanced stage of cancer is also related to higher risk of suicide ideation, suicide attempt, and completed suicide. A desire for hastened death has been reported as present in approximately 14% of patients in an advanced phase of cancer.[11]

Biological Risk Factors

Although current knowledge regarding the neurobiology of suicide is still insufficient, the biological psychiatry literature has focused on possible psychobiological concomitants of suicidal behavior. A series of studies have, for example, suggested that alterations in a number of neurobiological systems, including the serotonergic and noradrenergic systems, the hypothalamic-pituitary-adrenal axis, and immune dysregulation are associated with depression and suicidal behavior.[12,13] Altered functioning of these neurobiological systems may stem both from genetic causes and developmental causes, such as adversity in early life, which may have consequences in reducing the threshold of stress resistance in adulthood, as well as the interaction of early-life experiences of adversity and genetic vulnerability.[14] Inflammation may also play an important role in the pathophysiology of suicide, especially levels of some specific inflammatory cytokines. An increase of the serum concentrations of proinflammatory cytokines, such as tumor necrosis factor α, interferon γ, interleukin (IL)-1, and IL-6, have been found among suicide victims and attempters. With respect to this, the levels of IL-6 in the peripheral blood has been proposed as a biological suicide marker, while increased levels of IL-4 and IL-13 transcription in the orbitofrontal cortex of completed suicides have been suggested to affect neurobehavioral processes relevant to suicide.[15,16]

More recent data have also proposed, by using convergent functional genomics involving genes and immune and inflammatory responses, a universal predictive measure as a broad-spectrum predictor of suicide across psychiatric diagnoses.[17] From the clinical point of view, these variables are difficult to monitor in oncology, given the effects on the same neurobiological systems (including cytokines levels) determined by cancer and cancer treatment. However, exploration of early-life events and adversity, depressive episodes in the past, and a history of depression and suicide in the family may be further alerting elements in terms of psychobiological risk for suicide in cancer patients. See Box 4.1 for notable risk factors.

> **Box 4.1 Notable Risk Factors**
>
> - Family history of major depression and suicide (attempt or completed suicide)
> - Individual past history of depression and early adversity
> - Individual past history of suicide attempts
> - Preexisting psychiatric disorders, including alcohol/drug abuse
> - Current psychiatric disorders (major depression, serious mental illness)
> - Patient age (elderly at increased risk)
> - Living alone/social isolation
> - Male gender
> - Cancer type (lung, stomach, head, and neck) and stage (advanced)

Presenting Problems

Key Symptoms and Signs

All oncology staff need to be familiar with the key signs and symptoms that suggest increased suicide risk in their patients. Checking for clinical depression is an important preliminary step, and it is helpful if staff become familiar with basic assessment methods that can flag suicide risk. See Box 4.2 for details.

Expressing suicidal thoughts and intentions is an indicator of serious low mood and suicide risk. If in doubt, the clinician should arrange an urgent assessment by a mental health colleague as soon as possible; preferably within 24 hours. If a mental health professional is not available at the time the practitioner thinks the patient might be at risk, he or she should proceed with an appropriate assessment to determine mental health status.

It is helpful to differentiate active from passive suicidal thoughts: for example, (a) Active: "I want to die because this pain is terrible." (b) Passive: "As my quality of life has deteriorated, I'm ready to die when that time comes." (c) Active planning: "I will take an overdose of sedatives tonight after I've finished saying my family goodbyes." (d) Passive with no planning: "I accept dying, but won't need to do anything to hasten it. I hope that God takes me soon."

It is also helpful to identify the presence of mounting desperation and a highly lethal plan of action: for example, "Tell me the method you plan to

> **Box 4.2 Ascertain Suicide Plan**
>
> 🔍 *Key Questions:*
> - Does the patient have a clear suicide plan?
> - What would they do?
> - Under what circumstances would they carry out their plan?
> - How likely are they to carry it out?

use to end your life" or "Help me to understand how desperate you feel about this." A grave risk exists when a desperate patient is indicating a highly lethal plan, and immediate and constant containment by staff is required in this setting.

Key Problems

Managing a patient at risk of suicide often presents a need for immediate decision-making to keep patients safe from harm. Decisions made will depend on whether the patient is in a hospital/clinic as an inpatient or attending as an outpatient. In some instances, suicide risk may be reported by family members or carers, who need to be questioned on what has happened that leads them to consider the patient at risk. Actions taken then depend on which medical practitioner currently holds a *duty of care* for the patient—the oncologist, community physician, or psychiatrist, for example. Generally, if the patient is physically within a clinician's current duty of care (e.g., on-site in the clinic or ward), that person will have immediate responsibility for providing a *place of safety*. The most commonly employed strategy is to ask a personal care attendant or nurse to sit beside patients and accompany them to the toilet, so that their whereabouts are known at all times. Nonmedical oncology staff require a clear policy to follow if they have concerns about a cancer patient in their care.

Investigations and actions need to

- Clarify level of risk.
- Ascertain if the patient has capacity.
- Ascertain contributing factors, both medical and social.
- Determine if the patient needs to be moved, or can be moved, to a place of safety.
- Determine if the patient is a risk to others.
- Clarify whether security staff are available to help with restraint if needed.
- Clarify if the patient is known to mental health services and, if yes, clarify who to contact regarding further management.

A general sense of panic among oncology staff may be evident, but when handled with skill and calm, the situation should be controllable. While determining appropriate actions, safety measures should be in place so that patients and staff at the oncology center/clinic are not put at risk.

What if the patient attempts to leave the oncology clinic or ward?

Attempting to stop a patient at suicide risk from leaving the clinic or hospital is *inadvisable if there is any immediate risk of violence or aggression to staff or others*. In these circumstances, patients at risk of self-harm who are attempting to leave the hospital or clinic against medical/nursing advice should be allowed to do so, and the next step is to *immediately call hospital security staff, the emergency services or police*, who will detain the patient and take him or her to a place of safety, usually a mental health unit, where the patient may be detained for assessment by mental health professionals according to the law.

Be aware: once a patient has been assessed by a mental health professional to ascertain suicide risk, returning the patient to his or her cancer treatment center as soon as possible is a priority. There is little point in preventing a suicide attempt if the patient then becomes at risk due to serious disruption of the cancer treatment. For these reasons, oncology patients with suicidal thinking might be optimally accommodated on an inpatient oncology ward, with a personal care assistant or nurse stationed by their bed on a 24-hour roster until treatment reduces their suicide risk. If this is not practical, it is important that in circumstances where care of the patient is handed over (albeit temporarily) to a mental health professional, the latter must be provided with any information about the patient's oncology care that is relevant to keeping the patient safe.

Diagnostic Difficulties

There are several problems when dealing with patients with severe mental illness who develop cancer. The first relates to the tendency physicians have to minimize the clinical significance of physical complaints in patients with severe mental illness, a phenomenon called *diagnostic overshadowing*. This can indicate progression of an *underdiagnosed cancer* with a worsening of the patients' physical condition attributed inappropriately to the mental illness. Contrary to this, in some instances there can be overdiagnosis of clinical depression due to symptoms of cancer and cancer treatment (e.g., cachexia, sleep loss, fatigue, loss of appetite) being misattributed to depression. This makes it important to distinguish symptoms of clinical depression from cancer-related symptoms. *A thorough knowledge of the patient's current cancer care is important to making an accurate differential diagnosis of depression and suicide risk.*

Occasionally profound fatigue may be confused as a symptom of clinical depression. It is helpful to assess cancer patients in order to distinguish depression-related fatigue symptoms. In general, patients with fatigue are usually able to derive some pleasure from activities that they normally enjoy, and late afternoon is often the most difficult time, while, typically, depressed patients are unable to enjoy usual things (anhedonia) and have a sense of hopelessness. Morning is often the most difficult time with depressed cancer patients being unable to motivate themselves. (See chapter 2 for guidelines on distinguishing cancer-related fatigue symptoms from depression.)

Investigations for Key Differential Diagnosis

It is sometimes difficult to distinguish passive expressions of suicidal intention made within the context of normal sadness and disease progression toward normal dying from real threats of self-harm. Elicit whether the patient has a clear plan and the circumstances in which he or she would self-harm and how. This should help to establish the seriousness of a threat of self-harm or suicide in the patient. Follow the steps in Box 4.2 to ascertain if the patient has a suicide plan.

Assessment

While there are a number of paper-and-pencil tests that can assist staff in screening patients for mental health problems, the most accurate, reliable, and comprehensive methods are best applied within the context of a clinical diagnostic interview such as a mental status examination.

Questionnaires can provide a brief screening method to indicate if a clinical interview is required. Questionnaires have varying false positive and negative rates, and clinical management of suicide risk should never be based on questionnaire assessments alone.

Many cancer professionals are apprehensive about making an interview-based mental status examination given lack of time or skill. However, key questions can be asked quickly and may save time if applied skillfully. These skills are usually within the capacity of most cancer professionals. For example, clinicians can ask patients, "How does life seem to you at this point?" or "Have you ever felt that life was not worth living?" or "Did you ever wish you could go to sleep and just not wake up?" They should focus on the nature, frequency, extent, and timing of suicidal thoughts and consider the patient's interpersonal, situational, and symptomatic context, as well as speak with family members or friends to determine whether they have observed unusual behaviors (e.g., recent purchase of a gun) or are privy to thoughts that suggest suicidal ideation. All of these skills can be part of the armamentarium of health care professionals. See the assessment tool in Box 4.3.

> **Box 4.3 Assessment Tool**
>
> Core presenting symptoms associated with suicidal thinking:
> - Hopelessness/helplessness
> - Meaninglessness/bleak view of the future/cannot see a future
> - Shame at predicament or behavior
> - Guilt feelings or feelings of worthlessness
> - Anhedonia (loss of interest/inability to enjoy usual things)
> - Depressed mood/flatness of affect/pervasive sadness
> - Diurnal variation in mood (worse in mornings)
> - Frequent weepiness (crying may be normal so check context and appropriateness)
> - Sleep disturbance/memory and concentration problems/loss of interest in food/ fatigue (not obviously disease-related)
> - Check duration and intensity of symptoms (duration of two weeks or more)

Clinical Management

Having established there is risk of suicide, the following actions in this checklist are helpful.

Check [✓] the following:

☐ Is the patient in your duty of care?

☐ Is there any immediate risk of self-harm?

☐ Are patient's medications controlled to avoid use for self-harm?

- ☐ Does the patient have any access to other means of self-harm?
- ☐ Are any medical symptoms contributing?
- ☐ Is the patient in a safe environment?

Consider using the steps described in Box 4.4 for inpatient management.

> **Box 4.4 Inpatient Management**
>
> ✓ Place the patient on 1:1 observation and review the need for continuing observation after 24 hours.
> ✓ All staff taking an observational role should be briefed regarding what to do if the patient attempts to leave their care or is seen to be self-harming.
> ✓ Enter details of the care plan into medical (and nursing) notes, including any record/details of patient *advance directive/decisions*.
> ✓ Decide who will be responsible for reviewing the patient.
> ✓ Indicate the next review date/time, and record this in the medical and nursing notes.
> ✓ Seek urgent advice and assessment from the oncology mental health team.

Pharmacological Options

The psychopharmacological treatment of the underlying psychiatric illness is the most effective antisuicide approach for patients with psychiatric disorders showing suicidal thoughts or behaviors (see also chapter 5). In depression, the evidence that antidepressant (AD) treatments decrease suicide risk or the likelihood of a suicide attempt is mixed or inconclusive in the short term. It is, however, essential that the treatment for depression is organized in agreement with accepted psychopharmacology guidelines in three phases: acute, continuation, and maintenance (if appropriate).

- The goals of the acute phase (three to four weeks) are to achieve remission (resolution of all symptoms) and restore functioning.
- The goal of the continuation phase (six months following full remission of the acute episode) is sustained remission, since failure to achieve complete remission (recovery) has major adverse consequences, including sustained risk of suicide.
- If the risk for recurrence is low, treatment should be gradually tapered over a period of one to three months, while if the risk of recurrence is high, long-term treatment maintenance is necessary for a minimum of three to five years. (See Krupfer in the Further Reading section.)

Some key management principles include the following.

- When prescribing ADs, it is always advisable to select a drug with a low risk of lethality on acute overdose, such as a selective serotonin reuptake inhibitor (SSRI) or other newer ADs (e.g., mirtazapine, venlafaxine) and to prescribe conservative quantities (see Box 4.5).
- Among patients with bipolar disorders or mixed major mood disorders, long-term lithium treatment has been shown to markedly reduce (approximately 80%) the risk of suicide attempts and of completed suicides.

> **Box 4.5 Efficacy and Safety of Psychotropic Drugs in the Treatment of Major Psychiatric Disorders in Oncology, Considering the Possible Risk of Suicide**
>
> Monitor constantly suicide ideation in the acute phase of treatment.
>
> *Tricyclics*
> Potentially fatal in overdose
>
> *Serotonin Reuptake Inhibitors (SSRIs)*
> Low risk of death in overdose
>
> *Serotonin and Norepinephrine Reuptake Inhibitor (SNRIs)*
>
> *Norepinephrine and Dopamine Reuptake Inhibitors (NRIs)*
> Potentially fatal in overdose
>
> *Antipsychotics*
> Potentially fatal in overdose
>
> Adapted, modified, and expanded from Grassi et al. (2014). See Further Reading.

- Among patients with schizophrenia, clozapine has been reported to have a specific antisuicide effect and it is the first FDA-approved medication with this indication.
- Some data have been collected on the use of other antipsychotic drugs in reducing suicide risk, such as olanzapine or quetiapine in combination with a mood-stabilizing agent.
- Treatment of psychological symptoms possibly accompanying suicidal ideation, such as severe insomnia, agitation, and marked anxiety, is necessary by using medications that can be effective on these symptoms, such as benzodiazepines, trazodone, low doses of some second-generation antipsychotics (e.g., quetiapine), and some anticonvulsants, such as gabapentin. (See also chapter 5.)

Psychotherapeutic Options

Psychotherapy has an important role in the treatment of patients reporting suicidal ideation or suicidal behaviors, with a substantial body of evidence supporting the efficacy of psychotherapeutic intervention in the treatment of specific disorders, such as major depressive disorder and borderline personality disorder, which are associated with increased suicide risk. Among these interventions, cognitive behavioral therapy is frequently used alongside psycho-pharmacological treatment. *All psychotherapies should preferably be delivered by an appropriately training professional, often a recognized mental health professional* (e.g., counselor, oncology nurse consultant with specialist mental health training, mental health nurse, social worker, clinical or health psychologist, psychiatrist, psychotherapist). For more details on psychotherapy techniques to use with cancer patients see chapter 2 and the *Handbook of Psychotherapy in Cancer Care* (Watson and Kissane in Further Reading).

Case Study

An Integrated Psychopharmacological Approach

Teresa is a 63-year-old woman working as a housewife. She lives with her husband. Two years ago, she was diagnosed with ovarian cancer and underwent surgery, followed by chemotherapy and radiotherapy. Things went well until the last month, when she started to complain of weakness, loss of appetite and weight loss, and a constant pain at the site of operation and in the abdomen. She is not able to do her job at home and spends most of the time in a bed or a chair. Her husband takes her to the general practitioner who, suspecting a possible recurrence of cancer, asks for a series of examinations, including an oncological consultation. At the consultation with the oncologist, an admission to the hospital to accelerate the tests is arranged. During one of the first rounds, the oncologist asks for possible problems and also administers the NCCN Distress Thermometer (DT) and the problem list. The DT score is 8, and many problems are indicated by Teresa, including depression and anxiety. This opens a fruitful conversation with the oncologist, who requests a psychiatric consultation with the hospital psycho-oncology service. All the other test results (blood tests, CT scan, MRI, PET) are negative. In the meeting with the psychiatrist that Teresa also accepted, some important elements emerge.

The patient has been living for 37 years with a man whom she feels is not talkative, very unemotional, not supportive, and only interested in "his things," although she admits he is worried about Teresa's health conditions. Teresa recently had a number of stressful events, including the divorce of her daughter four months ago, which created many problems in the family. In the past, Theresa suffered from a depressive episode after the death of her mother (also of cancer). This episode went undiagnosed and untreated. At the clinical examination, Teresa is anxious. She describes a "sense of not having feelings anymore," with pervasive thinking about no future possible, emptiness, hopelessness, and helplessness. She is also focused on her abdominal pain, worrying her cancer may come back, despite the negative laboratory and medical tests. Theresa thinks that if her pain goes on, life is not worthwhile anymore and she is better off dead. This suicidal ideation increased in the last week, but she did not tell anyone. There is not a completely structured plan about how to die, but Teresa has thought of overdosing herself with the medications she and her husband have at home (including antihypertensive agents, anticoagulants, and insulin her husband takes for diabetes) or to drown herself in the river near the town. She feels worse in the morning and a little better in the evening. Night is considered a relief, since it is the only time she does not think of or feel the pain. Each morning is "just the beginning of a new nightmare."

A diagnosis of recurrent major depression is formulated and an integrated psychopharmacological approach is commenced (venlafaxine 37.5mg, titrated at 75–102.5–150 mg a day; alprazolam 0.5 mg three times a day) during her stay in the oncology ward, with psychiatry/psycho-oncology consultations on a daily basis. A meeting with the husband and the daughter is called to gain more details about the family situation and to organize a plan for discharge, with referral to the outpatient psycho-oncology service.

Patient Capacity Issues in Management of Self-Harm Risk

The question of a patient's capacity is underpinned by five key principles.

- There is a *presumption of capacity* until proven otherwise. Therefore the evidence needs to prove they *do not* have capacity.
- Individuals have the right to be *supported* in making their own decisions.
- Individuals retain the right to make what might be seen as unwise or eccentric decisions *while still having capacity*.
- The principle of *"best interests"* must be followed. Anything done for, or on behalf of, people without capacity must be in their best interests.
- The *least restrictive intervention* in terms of basic rights and freedoms must be used. (See Box 4.6.)

Box 4.6 Patients' Rights within the Law

General principle of medical law: "Every human being of adult years and sound mind has a right to determine what shall be done with his own body."
Justice Cardozo, New York (1914)

Does the patient lack capacity? Is the patient of sound mind?

Medical practitioners usually have to indicate they are providing the necessary support to facilitate capacity. Thus they must *document everything clearly in the medical notes and seek a second opinion if in doubt*. In some countries, an independent second opinion is required if ascertainment of capacity is undertaken. Practitioners must be familiar with their country's laws regarding assessment of capacity in patients with serious mental health problems being treated for cancer. They should seek a second opinion from a mental health colleague if lack of capacity appears to be linked to serious mental illness. In many countries, medical practitioners take responsibility for establishing *if the patient lacks capacity*. In some countries, two medical practitioners are required to make independent assessments to establish consensus that the patient lacks capacity. Clinicians must follow known legal requirements for establishing whether a patient lacks capacity. What actions follow will be determined by the soundness of the clinical assessment of capacity.

The importance of staff safety

Where patients lack capacity, well-informed and confident staff are more likely to manage their own and the patient's safety effectively. While laws regarding compulsory detention under a mental health policy may differ from country to country, it is important to take steps within one's legal framework that aim to—if necessary—bring the patient to a place of safety (i.e., a mental health unit or cancer unit with appropriate facilities to manage suicide risk). See Box 4.7 for important actions to take when a patient is detained for emergency psychiatric treatment.

The confused patient

Where capacity issues are due to patient confusion, this is often caused by medical/physical factors. Tests to clarify the cause of confusion or agitation may take some time. Therefore, where possible, provide sedation to the patient.

> **Box 4.7 Detention for Emergency Psychiatric Treatment**
>
> ⚗ *Key Message*
> If a patient is detained for a mental health assessment and emergency psychiatric treatment:
> - It is important for oncology staff to liaise with the acute psychiatric emergency services to clarify the patient's cancer treatment status and deal with any possible cancer treatment–related issues.
> - Emergency services personnel need to know what medications have been recorded in the medical notes for the patient so they can be aware of any drug interactions and how oncology medication history may impact their management of an acute psychiatric episode linked to suicide risk.

Sedate only if there is risk to the safety of the patient or others
Speaking quietly and calmly to the patient helps. Where possible, clinicians should offer patients who place themselves and others at risk the choice of oral or IV medication to help them feel less confused and calm. Staff confronted with a confused patient may feel out of their depth and unable to cope. Providing staff with clear instructions helps. The lead clinician should take responsibility for providing instructions to staff. Immediate investigations should take place to establish the cause of confusion in patients. *All staff involved in the confused patient's care should have access to instructions, entered into the medical and nursing notes, about whom to contact if the patient deteriorates and what steps to take to ensure patient and staff safety.*

Use of restraint
Staff required to restrain a patient must have appropriate training. A four-point physical restraint is the most commonly used (for arms and legs).

Establish: Is the patient neutropenic? Is the patient frail? Does the patient have any surgical or medical contra-indications to the use of restraint? Clinicians must be clear about the legal requirements involving use of restraint, who may authorize the use of restraint, and when this must be reviewed. They should always do what is in the patient's best interest. Following the actions described in Box 4.8 relating to sedation and restraint safety issues will help.

> **Box 4.8 Sedation and Restraint Safety Issues**
>
> ⚗ *Key Message*
> - Always seek help from colleagues and/or security staff if intending to sedate patients without their consent.
> - Be aware that inappropriate use of restraint and sedation in patients with capacity may be considered a criminal offence in some countries.

The unconscious patient

When a patient is unconscious and it is suspected or evident that self-harm is the cause of unconsciousness, then the practitioner should follow these guidelines:

- Determine if the patient needs to be transferred to the emergency room.
- Act with urgency in this situation.
- Check if anyone was with the patient just prior to him or her losing consciousness and ascertain if there is information on the exact cause of unconsciousness.

Unconscious patients, by most legal guidelines, *are lacking in capacity*. The clinician must then act in the patient's best interests. All actions must be subsequently clearly documented in medical notes and preferably checked by a second medical practitioner. If the patient dies in a medical practitioner's care as a result of suicide, the practitioner is usually asked to "make a deposition," giving an account of events and their actions; in most cases, this deposition will go to a coroners court or a similar court depending on the country laws. *Therefore, as soon as possible, all events and actions taken must be recorded.*

Delirium

Sometimes confusion arises about the management of patients with delirium as they may place themselves at risk. Bizarre behaviors sometimes lead to a misdiagnosis of mental illness. Delirium is a clinical syndrome characterized by a disturbance of arousal, attention, perception, and other cognitive domains, which tends to have a fluctuating course. Onset is usually (not always) acute. It can include any of the following, which may be misinterpreted as evidence of mental illness rather than physical disequilibrium:

- Changed level of arousal (e.g., drowsy or agitated) and mood change, including dysphoria/euphoria, fear, anxiety, crying, laughing, being labile, and/or constricted emotions.
- Disordered thoughts and thought content or perceptual disorganization such as hallucinations.
- Lack of insight and judgment and disturbances in cognitive domains and sleep-wake cycles, along with psychomotor changes, including agitation.

Aetiology is linked to medication side effects (e.g., intoxication, withdrawal syndromes), postoperative states, hypoxia or hypercapnia, metabolic derangements, head trauma, infections/fever, and sleep and sensory deprivation. The patient with delirium may exhibit disturbed behavior (e.g., aggression, combativeness, noncompliance with treatment) and confusion (e.g., wandering, disorientation, nighttime change, absconding from the ward) with reported hallucinations. There are issues relating to lack of capacity and ability to consent. Patients with delirium may place themselves at risk of self-harm; however, there is usually an underlying medical aetiology, and medical rather than psychiatric management is primary.

While sedation and antipsychotic medication may be the first line of treatment, these management strategies can be delivered by oncology professionals, with a second opinion from a psychiatrist as required. Like acute depressive episodes and suicidal intentions, delirium needs to be *treated as an emergency* in order to keep the patient and others safe from harm.

> **Box 4.9 At-Risk Patients with Suicidal Thoughts in the Community**
>
> ⚠ *Warning*
> - If in doubt about patient safety—call emergency services.
> - Inform the community physician and request an urgent assessment/follow-up by a community mental health professional.
> - Is compulsory admission required to manage acute risk (within the appropriate mental health laws)? Liaise with the community psychiatric emergency team.

Patients in the community
If suicidal thoughts are expressed by someone in the community, the actions described in Box 4.9 will prove helpful.

Professional Issues and Service Implementation

Recording and Communicating

Practitioners should provide a complete and clear written record in the appropriate medical notes of any events and actions taken. They must be familiar with their *legal obligations* regarding recording of a patient's self-harm incident and must always review actions as soon as possible with a mental health colleague. Details of any psychotropic medications administered and whether this was with, or without, patient consent should be recorded, and a management plan for nursing and medical staff to follow should be considered, as well as whether a psychiatric opinion has been requested, with appropriate details recorded.

Legal Responsibilities

Any medical management plan for suicide risk will be linked to legal requirements. If intending to detain a patient on the grounds of mental health problems contributing to suicide risk, clinicians must be familiar with the law or, at the very least, seek advice and guidance from a mental health professional.

Ethical Dilemmas

Confidentiality
Health professionals have a duty of care that requires they communicate information to other practitioners if they believe the information-sharing is in the patient's best interest. When patients indicate they may place themselves at harm and list the circumstances in which they would self-harm, mental health professionals should inform the patient that, as a duty of care, *they must share this information with oncology colleagues so that the best treatment and care possible can be provided to the patient.*

Mental health professionals given confidential information by their patients with cancer that is about a third party (e.g., "my son has schizophrenia") are not at liberty to share this information with others unless they believe their patient or others may be put at risk. If a patient seen by mental health professionals admits an intention to harm a health-care professional/colleague under some circumstances (e.g., "my husband has promised to shoot the surgeon if I die during the cancer operation"), the professional has a duty to break patient confidentiality to protect the colleague at risk.

Advanced directives

Ethical dilemmas about suicide attempts can arise if there is a recorded advance decision or advanced directive about nonresuscitation. Patients who have made a suicide attempt that needs to be treated in order to ensure their safety may have a recorded advanced directive, but the clinician would be obliged to act in the patient's best interests, in case the patient's judgement was impaired at the time of the suicide attempt. If a depressed patient attempts suicide, his or her judgement may have been impaired at the time of this action, and resuscitation would be obligatory under the codes of most countries, irrespective of an advanced directive.

Known mental illness

Patients who attempt suicide are considered to lack capacity under the laws of many countries and may be treated without consent under the appropriate sections of the mental health laws. If an oncology professional is unfamiliar with the mental health laws, *then an urgent second opinion from a mental health professional should be requested*, including emergency transfer of the patient without consent to an appropriate mental health unit.

Policies and Protocols

All oncology treatment centers should develop a policy about the management of suicide risk in their patients. Such policy documents need to be checked by a lawyer for legal correctness and against country practice guidelines as specified in law. Policy documents should be easily accessible to staff involved in the care of cancer patients.

The mortality review process in the case of a patient's death due to suicide should be laid out as a clear protocol for quality assurance purposes. All therapists need to work to an agreed policy on how to deal with psychiatric emergencies, and procedures will vary depending on the context and country in which one is based. Box 4.10 provides suggestions on management policies.

A flow-chart of actions is set out in Figure 4.1.

Box 4.10 Management Policies

- All oncology units should have an agreed policy for managing suicide risk both for inpatients and outpatients.
- This policy document should be easily accessible for reference by clinical staff, including nursing staff.
- The policy should preferably provide a responsibilities flowchart indicating who takes what actions, and all clinical staff should know how to access this information. Copies should be kept in ward offices as well as on clinical service computer systems and regularly used staff-only areas, as appropriate.

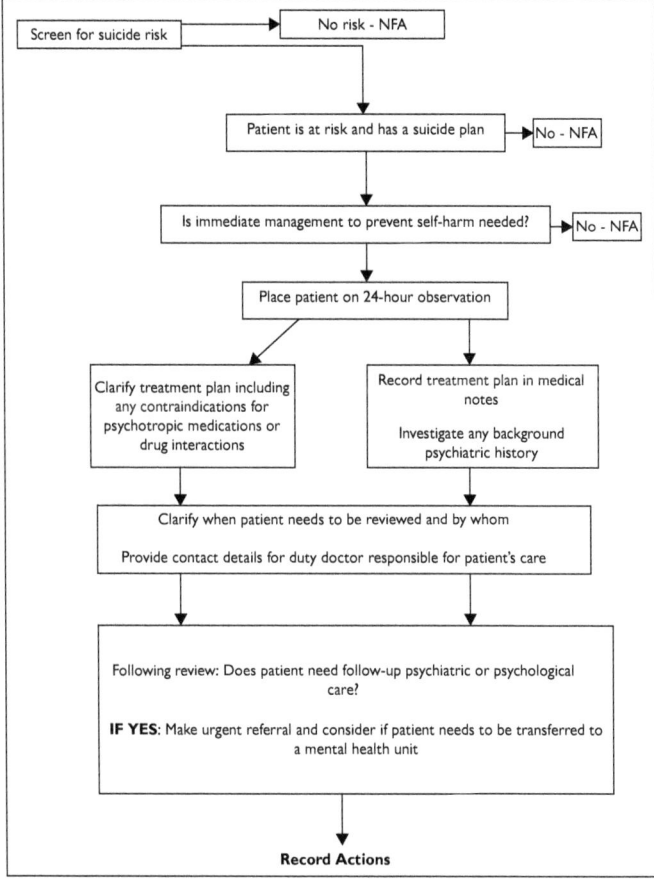

Figure 4.1. Suicide Risk Management Flowchart (NFA = no further action)

Teams and Supervision

The ideal model is a multidisciplinary team that meets and reviews patients regularly and has a nominated mental health professional from whom opinions and advice can be sought as required. While resources may be limited in terms of access to supervision by a mental health professional, regular peer supervision should be the standard applied. This may include weekly team meetings and/or regular multidisciplinary meetings, where the review of patient care always includes the question of whether there is knowledge of the patient needing mental health care alongside cancer care.

References

1. Misono S, Weiss NS, Fann JR, Redman M, Yueh B. Incidence of suicide in persons with cancer. *J Clin Oncol*. 2008;26(29):4731–4738.

2. Smailyte G, Jasilionis D, Kaceniene A, Krilaviciute A, Ambrozaitiene D, Stankuniene V. Suicides among cancer patients in Lithuania: a population-based census-linked study. *Cancer Epidemiol*. 2013 Oct;37(5):714–718.

3. Miller M, Mogun H, Azrael D, Hempstead K, Solomon DH. Cancer and the risk of suicide in older Americans. *J Clin Oncol*. 2008;26(29):4720–4724.

4. Walker J, Hansen CH, Butcher I., et al. Thoughts of death and suicide reported by cancer patients who endorsed the "suicidal thoughts" item of the PHQ-9 during routine screening for depression. *Psychosomatics*. 2011;52(5):424–427.

5. Robson A, Scrutton F, Wilkinson L, MacLeod F. The risk of suicide in cancer patients: a review of the literature. *Psychooncology* 2010;19(12):1250–1258.

6. Spoletini I, Gianni W, Caltagirone C, Madaio R, Repetto L, Spalletta G. Suicide and cancer: where do we go from here? *Crit Rev Oncol Hematol*. 2011 Jun;78(3):206–219.

7. Anguiano L, Mayer DK, Piven ML, Rosenstein D. A literature review of suicide in cancer patients. *Cancer Nurs*. 2012 Jul-Aug;35(4):E14–E26.

8. Fang F, Fall K, Mittleman MA, et al. Suicide and cardiovascular death after a cancer diagnosis. *N Engl J Med*. 2012;366(14):1310–1318.

9. Choi YN, Kim YA, Yun YH, et al. (2014). Suicide ideation in stomach cancer survivors and possible risk factors. *Support Care Cancer*. 2014;22:331–337.

10. Ahn MH, Park S, Lee HB, et al. Suicide in cancer patients within the first year of diagnosis. *Psychooncology*. 2014;24(5):601–607. doi:10.1002/pon.3705

11. Kelly B, Burnett P, Pelusi D, et al. Factors associated with the wish to hasten death: a study of patients with terminal illness. *Psychol Med*. 2003;33(1):75–81.

12. Mann JJ, Currier DM. Stress, genetics and epigenetic effects on the neurobiology of suicidal behavior and depression. *Eur Psychiatry*. 2010 Jun;25(5):268–271.

13. Gançana L, Oquendo MA, Tyrka AR, Cisneros-Trujillo S, Mann JJ, Sublette ME. The role of cytokines in the pathophysiology of suicidal behavior. *Psychoneuroendocrinology*. 2016 Jan;63:296–310.

14. Labonte B, Turecki G. The epigenetics of suicide: explaining the biological effects of early life environmental adversity. *Arch Suicide Res*. 2010;14(4):291–231.

15. Serafini G, Pompili M, Seretti ME, et al. The role of inflammatory cytokines in suicidal behavior: a systematic review. *Eur Neuropsychopharmacol*. 2013;23:1672–1686.

16. Miná VAL, Lacerda-Pinheiro SF, Maia LC, et al. The influence of inflammatory cytokines in physiopathology of suicidal behavior. *J Affect Disord*. 2015;172:219–230.

17. Niculescu AB, Levey DF, Phalen PL, et al. Understanding and predicting suicidality using a combined genomic and clinical risk assessment approach. *Mol Psychiatr*. 2015;20(11):1266–2385.

Further Reading

American Psychiatric Association. *Assessing and Treating Suicidal Behaviors: A Quick Reference Guide*. Washington, DC: American Psychiatric Association; 2003.

American Psychiatric Association. *Practice Guideline for the Assessment and Treatment of Patients with Suicidal Behaviors*. Washington, DC: American Psychiatric Association; 2003.

Provides detailed practice guidelines for reference.

Kupfer DJ. The pharmacological management of depression. *Dialogues Clin Neurosci*. 2005;7:191–205.

Provides detailed information on use of medications to treat depression.

Watson M, Kissane D. *Handbook of Psychotherapy in Cancer Care*. London: John Wiley; 2011.

Explains detailed models of psychotherapy and how they are applied in cancer care.

Chapter Quiz

1. The rate of completed suicides in cancer patients is
   A. the same as in the general population.
   B. higher than in patients with renal disease.
   C. about 1.5 times higher than that of the general population.
   D. lower than that of the general population.
   E. about three times higher than that of the general population.

2. A patient is in your neighborhood and telephones you to say he is going to kill himself. What should you do?
   A. Try to talk the patient out of it.
   B. Give the patient an appointment to come and see you.
   C. Ask what the patient would do, when and how.
   E. Ask the patient to speak to a friend to get some help.

3. A patient is in the clinic and tells a nurse that she is going to take a bottle of Paracetamol. What should you do?
   A. Tell the nurse to try to talk the patient out of it.
   B. Give the patient an appointment to come and see you later that day.
   C. See the patient as a priority, treating this as an emergency, and assess whether she is depressed.
   D. Demand the patient hand over the bottle of Paracetamol and threaten to detain her at the hospital.

4. The main risk factors for suicide to be assessed when evaluating cancer patients are
   A. social and stressful factors (e.g., separation, divorce, unemployment).
   B. current psychiatric disorder (including depression).
   C. suicide ideation.
   D. disability and physical symptoms secondary to the disease or treatment.
   E. all the above.

Chapter 5

Psychopharmacologic Management of Anxiety and Depression

Madeline Li, Joshua Rosenblat, and Gary Rodin

Learning Objectives

After reading this chapter, the clinician will be able to
1. Understand the importance of the identification and effective treatment of depression and anxiety in cancer settings.
2. Appreciate the continuum of distress from a normative response of sadness or worry to pathological depression or anxiety.
3. Review the indications and contraindications for pharmacological management of depression and anxiety in cancer settings.
4. Consider adverse effects and drug–drug interactions when selecting the most appropriate medication to treat depression and/or anxiety.
5. Explore the application of pharmacological management algorithms to specific case examples of depression and anxiety disorders.

Background Evidence

Depression and anxiety are extremely common in patients with cancer, with approximately 16% suffering from major depression and 10% from anxiety disorders at any one time.[1] Effective management of these symptoms is important, as they are associated with lower quality of life, reduced survival rates, prolonged hospital stays, physical distress, poorer treatment compliance, increased suicidal thoughts, and completed suicide.[2]

Appropriate selection of interventions for depression or anxiety requires an understanding of the nature and severity of the symptoms. Mild nonpathological symptoms should be distinguished from more severe symptoms that may meet criteria for a *Diagnostic and Statistical Manual of Mental Disorders* (fifth edition; DSM-5)–defined mood or anxiety disorder (Table 5.1).

While a diagnosis of cancer often precipitates a patient's *first* major depressive episode, the appearance of an anxiety disorder is more likely due to a reactivation of a preexisting disorder rather than the first presentation of a new anxiety disorder.[3] The diagnostic features of select anxiety disorders

Table 5.1 Psychological and Diagnostic Features on the Continuum of Distress

Normal Sadness	Subthreshold Disorders	DSM-5 Depressive Disorders
• Maintains intimacy and connection • Believes that things will get better • Can enjoy happy memories • Sense of self-worth fluctuates with thoughts of cancer • Looks forward to the future • Retains capacity for pleasure • Maintains will to live	• Low mood presentation similar to major depression but not meeting full criteria for symptom number or duration • May be transient and self-limited, including mood episodes lasting < 2 weeks • Includes persistent depressive disorder if > 2 years duration	• Feels isolated • Feeling of permanence • Excessive guilt and regret • Self-critical ruminations/loathing • Constant, pervasive, and nonreactive sadness • Sense of hopelessness • Loss of interest in activities • Suicidal thoughts/behavior • Meets diagnostic criteria for major depression

Normal Worries	Subthreshold Disorders	DSM-5 Anxiety Disorders
• Mild worries calmed with support and information • Transient anxiety that fluctuates with cancer-related events • Typical cancer-specific worries that settle over weeks/months • Maintains balanced perspective on worries, effective coping skills • Anxiety motivates treatment compliance • Only occasional physical symptoms of fatigue, poor sleep, appetite, or concentration • No panic attacks	• High levels of realistic worry, needs repeated reassurance • Frequent anxiety but can be distracted and sometimes not think about worries • Cancer-related worries that do not resolve over time • Focuses on negatives but can still see positives • Difficulty engaging in treatment but does attend • Physical symptoms present more often than not, more severe than expected for cancer stage and treatment • Occasional panic attacks triggered by specific thoughts or situations	• Disproportionate worry, unresponsive to reassurance • Constant worry, intrusive thoughts that are difficult to control • Unfocused anxiety, extending to multiple issues besides cancer • Catastrophizes, sees only worst-case scenarios • Unable to make decisions or engage in cancer treatment • Persistent and intractable physical symptoms, not relieved by usual supportive measures • Frequent panic attacks, often untriggered • Meets diagnostic criteria for a DSM-5 anxiety disorder

Note: DSM-5: *Diagnostic and Statistical Manual of Mental Disorders* (5th ed.; American Psychiatric Association, 2013).

Adapted with permission from Li, M, Kennedy EB, Byrne N, et al. The management of depression in patients with cancer: a quality initiative of the Program in Evidence-Based Care (PEBC), Cancer Care Ontario (CCO). Guideline #19-4. Toronto: Cancer Care Ontario, May 2015.

seen in cancer patients and how they may be manifest are summarized in chapter 1. However, the DSM-5 category that most closely fits the typical presentation of severe anxiety in cancer patients is unspecified anxiety disorder, defined as "clinically significant distress or impairment in social, occupational, or other important areas of functioning predominate but do not meet the full criteria for any of the disorders in the anxiety disorders diagnostic class."[4, p. 233] Symptoms of anxiety may heighten motivation to seek or continue with aversive cancer treatment but, when severe, may interfere with participation in cancer care. Key information is summarized in Box 5.1.

> **Box 5.1**
>
> Determining the nature and severity of depression and anxiety is required prior to initiating treatment. Pharmacologic treatments should generally be used only in conjunction with psychotherapeutic interventions. Pharmacologic management of depression and anxiety should be reserved for more severe symptoms.

Psychotherapeutic support is indicated throughout the trajectory of cancer to alleviate mild and more severe symptoms of anxiety and depression related to the disease and treatment and to address concerns such as those related to suffering, loss, uncertainty, dependency, and mortality (see chapters 1 and 2). Pharmacologic management should additionally be considered for more severe symptoms, the indication for which there is the most evidence.[5]

Randomized controlled trials assessing the efficacy of pharmacologic treatments of depression in cancer settings are limited, with unblinded case series still being reported.[6] Previous clinical trials have had significant limitations related to sample size, research design, and heterogeneity of depressive symptoms. Based on the trials assessing the efficacy of antidepressants, the pooled odds ratio suggests a small but statistically significant effect in the alleviation of depressive symptoms.[7]

The evidence base supporting pharmacologic treatment of anxiety in cancer is even more limited than that for depression.[8] Treatment studies have tended to include participants with both mild and severe anxiety and to be powered to assess anxiety only as a secondary outcome. Such trials are often too short for the anxiolytic effect to be evident, which may take longer to be evident than the antidepressant effect.

The conclusion reached in numerous systematic reviews and meta-analyses of treatment studies of anxiety and/or depression is that there is insufficient evidence to support the superiority of any particular drug or class of medications over another in cancer patients. The recommendations for treatment selection are, therefore, primarily based on evidence from studies in other medical populations and on expert consensus.[9,10] However, there are special considerations in cancer patients related to potential adverse effects and drug–drug interactions. This chapter provides recommendations and considerations for the pharmacologic management of moderate to severe forms of depression and anxiety in cancer patients.

General Principles of Pharmacologic Management for Anxiety and Depression in Cancer

Figure 5.1 provides an algorithm for the initial management of anxiety and depression in cancer patients, recognizing that these symptoms are frequently comorbid and respond to similar treatment approaches. The first step in management is a systematic approach to early detection. Screening for emotional distress is now widely recommended by most cancer care organizations and guidelines using any one of several validated anxiety and depression rating scales that are now available (see chapter 1). Such rating scales are also recommended to determine symptom severity and to monitor response to treatment over time. Following screening, appropriate clinical assessment is needed to confirm the presence of an anxiety (see chapter 1) or depressive (see chapter 2) disorder, to identify contributing or confounding conditions, and to assess the risk of suicide (see chapter 4).

Ruling out relevant disorders that may resemble depression or anxiety, such as hypoactive delirium, substance withdrawal, or cancer-related physical

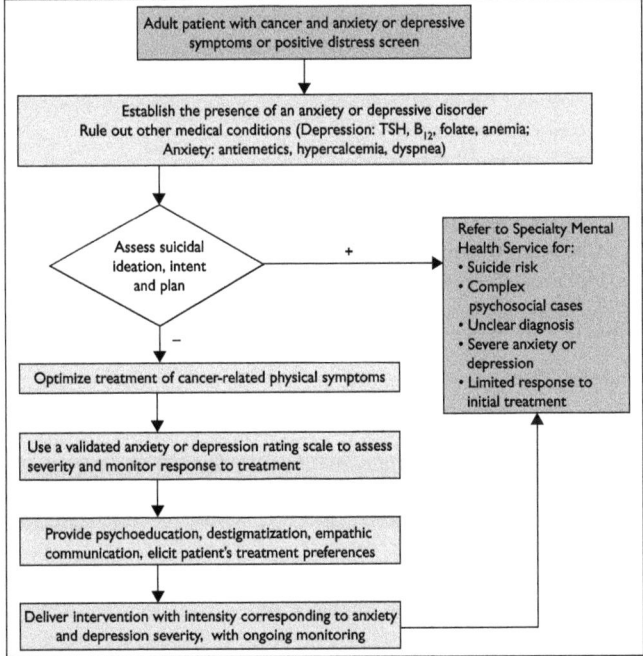

Figure 5.1. Algorithm for the initial management of anxiety and depression in cancer. Adapted with permission from Li, M, Kennedy EB, Byrne N, et al. The management of depression in patients with cancer: a quality initiative of the Program in Evidence-Based Care (PEBC), Cancer Care Ontario (CCO). Guideline #19-4. Toronto: Cancer Care Ontario; May 2015.

symptoms (e.g., fatigue, anorexia, and insomnia) is essential prior to selection of an intervention. Another key step in the management of depression and anxiety in cancer is ensuring the effective management of cancer-related physical symptoms.[11] If pain control is poor, pharmacologic management of mood and anxiety symptoms is likely to be ineffective. Therefore, assessment and optimization of cancer-related physical symptoms on an ongoing basis is an essential component of treatment. Prior to initiating an intervention, clinicians should also provide psychoeducation to inform patients about the benefit of treatment of severe anxiety or depression on cancer outcomes and to normalize and destigmatize symptoms by framing them as a consequence of cancer and its treatment. Treatment options should be discussed while encouraging participation of family members in the treatment plan. Patients' treatment preferences should be elicited. Most patients with cancer prefer psychological approaches. For more severe symptoms, pharmacotherapy may be required and may, in fact, enable to patients to better engage in psychological approaches. Further considerations in selecting pharmacotherapy for the treatment of depression and anxiety are presented in Box 5.2.

Box 5.2 When to Prescribe

1. Strong preference of the patient for medication approaches
2. Language, health, or other barriers that preclude participation in psychological therapies
3. A clear past history of an anxiety or depressive disorder that was responsive to medications
4. Severe anxiety or depression
5. Moderate anxiety or depression that
   - interferes with cancer care
   - persists after psychological interventions
6. Moderate depressive symptoms for at least two years
7. Transient moderate anxiety during stressful cancer-related events

Practical checklists are provided in Tool Kit 5.1 for how to initiate, maintain, and discontinue antidepressant medications. Prior to initiating a

Tool Kit 5.1 Practical Tools for Clinicians Prescribing an Antidepressant

Initiating an Antidepressant

☐ Screen for possible medical contributors to presenting conditions (e.g., TSH, vitamin B12), as well as substance use

☐ Start on lowest dose to minimize detrimental side effects and titrate up to therapeutic dose after first week

☐ Discuss potential detrimental side effects (particularly initial gastrointestinal upset, headache, or anxiety), which should resolve within the first week

(continued)

Tool Kit 5.1 Continued

- Explain that detrimental side effects occur before therapeutic benefit, which can take four to six weeks to reach full beneficial effect
- Advise that the risk of increased suicidality from antidepressants is small, most often associated with adolescents, and occurs early in the course of treatment
- Advise of the need to take medications daily and continue even after remission of depressive symptoms
- Counsel about potential discontinuation symptoms if medications are stopped abruptly
- Reassure patients that dependence or tolerance does not occur
- Discuss concerns related to antidepressants and potential increased suicidality

Maintaining an Antidepressant

- Provide support in first week when risk of nonadherence is greatest; follow up every two to four weeks until remission
- Monitor agitation, increased anxiety, and insomnia. Consider short-term benzodiazepine for initial symptoms, if required
- Assess response after three to four weeks at a therapeutic dose; increase dose if no response; switch medication if no response after six weeks
- Regularly monitor for changes in medical status and cancer treatments and adjust accordingly
- Continue at effective dose for at least six months after full remission
- Patients with a history of recurrent depression should be advised to continue maintenance treatment for at least two years or indefinitely

Discontinuing an Antidepressant

- Be aware that discontinuation syndromes (malaise, dizziness, agitation, headache, nausea, paresthesia) may occur with abrupt termination or missed doses at high dosage levels
- Recognize that discontinuation syndromes are more common with antidepressants with a shorter half-life (i.e., venlafaxine, paroxetine); they do not occur with fluoxetine
- Taper gradually over four weeks to minimize discontinuation syndromes; symptoms may be more prominent toward the end of the taper
- Advise that symptoms are usually mild and self-limiting over approximately one week
- If symptoms are severe, taper more slowly or consider switching to longer half-life SSRIs such as fluoxetine and then stopping
- Monitor for possible depression relapse over the next few months

medication, psychoeducation should be provided to fully inform patients of potential benefits and adverse effects. Further, the prescriber should explain that the common adverse effects, especially nausea, headache, and anxiety, are often time-limited and resolve after the first week of treatment. Patients should also be informed that there may be an increased risk of suicide that may occur before improvement in their depressed mood and that they should notify their caregivers if this effect occurs. A thorough explanation of potential adverse effects may help to prevent early treatment discontinuation. This includes clarification of the time lag of up to four to six weeks for the onset of the antidepressant effect. Such explanations are important both for informed consent and to increase adherence and the likelihood of symptom remission.

After an adequate course of antidepressant therapy has been completed, antidepressants may be continued or slowly tapered under the supervision of a clinician to prevent or reduce the occurrence of discontinuation syndromes. Symptoms of serotonin discontinuation include general malaise, dizziness, insomnia, headache, anxiety, agitation, and "shock-like" sensations, which generally resolve over the course of one to two weeks.

Attention to insomnia in anxiety or depression is also an important management consideration due to their bidirectional causal relationships, particularly during the lag period, until antidepressants take effect. After other potential causes of insomnia (e.g., steroid-induced insomnia) and adequate sleep hygiene have been addressed, insomnia may be addressed by selecting sedating antidepressants such as agomelatine, mirtazapine, or trazodone or through the short-term use of hypnotic agents, benzodiazepines, or sedating antipsychotics such as olanzapine or quetiapine (Table 5.2). Hypnotic agents should be tried first, due to their relatively lower potential for tolerance and withdrawal compared to benzodiazepines and lesser risk for drug interactions and fewer side effects compared to antipsychotics.

Pharmacologic Management of Depression in Cancer

Common Medication Classes Used in the Treatment of Major Depression

Table 5.2 also provides a comprehensive list of the more commonly used pharmacologic options to treat depression in cancer. Some, such as the monoamine oxidase inhibitors, are typically avoided because other medications with less toxicity and less interaction with medications commonly used in oncology are now available. Experimental therapies emerging for use in psychiatric populations, and alternative therapies frequently used by cancer patients, but are not discussed here because evidence to support their use is too limited. The more commonly used classes of medication are described here. (See Table 5.3.)

Selective serotonin reuptake inhibitors
Selective serotonin reuptake inhibitors (SSRIs) are the first choice in the treatment of major depression in cancer. While their efficacy is not greater than

Table 5.2 Psychotropics for the Management of Anxiety and Depression

Drugs	CYP450[a]	Common Side Effects	Cautions
Selective Serotonin Reuptake Inhibitors			
Citalopram	Strong 2D6/3A4	Initiating—GI upset, headache, dizziness, anxiety	• Citalopram/escitalopram QTc interval prolongation at high doses
Escitalopram	Strong 2D6	Longer term—sweating, sexual dysfunction, tremor, bruxism, weight gain	• Paroxetine has strong discontinuation syndrome
Sertraline	Moderate 2D6/1A2/3A4		• Risk of GI bleeding, hyponatremia, decreased bone density
Fluoxetine			
Paroxetine			
Fluvoxamine			
Mixed Action Reuptake Inhibitors (serotonin, norepinephrine, dopamine)			
Venlafaxine Desvenlafaxine	Moderate 2D6	GI upset, headache, dizziness, anxiety on initiation	• Venlafaxine discontinuation syndrome and hypertension risk
Duloxetine Milnacipran (SNRI)		Sweating, sexual dysfunction, constipation	• Duloxetine dose-dependent hepatotoxicity
Bupropion (NDRI)	Strong 2D6	Agitation	Seizure risk at high doses
Reboxetine (NRI)		Insomnia, sweating, dizziness, tachycardia	Caution in comorbid cardiac disease
Atypical Antidepressants			
Mirtazapine (NaSSA)		Sedation, weight gain, dry mouth, constipation	Rarely, reversible neutropenia
Agomelatine (Melatonin analog[b])	1A2 substrate	Mild nausea, dizziness, headache, somnolence	Caution in renal or hepatic impairment
Trazodone (SARI)		Sedation, dizziness, hypotension, GI distress, dry mouth, headache, rare priapism	More commonly used as a sleep aid due to intolerable sedation at therapeutic antidepressant doses
Vilazodone (SPARI)		GI upset, headache, dizziness, anxiety on initiation	May decrease the seizure threshold
Vortioxetine (SMS)		Nausea, vomiting, constipation, headache, sexual dysfunction	Gradual initiation due to increased GI intolerability

(continued)

Table 5.2 Continued

Drugs	CYP450[a]	Common Side Effects	Cautions
Buspirone (5-HT1A agonist)	3A4 substrate	Dizziness, headache, nausea, restlessness, somnolence.	Caution in hepatic or renal impairment
Tricyclic Antidepressants			
Amitriptyline Imipramine Nortriptyline Desipramine Lofepramine	3A4, 2D6, 1A2 substrate	Sedation, constipation, urinary retention, confusion, dry mouth, orthostatic hypotension, tachycardia	• High toxicity in overdose • 3° amines (amitriptyline, imipramine) less tolerable • Risk of QTc prolongation • May lower seizure threshold
Monoamine Oxidase Inhibitors			
Phenelzine Tranylcypromine Moclobemide	Moderate 2C19	Agitation, anxiety, insomnia, weakness, dizziness, hypotension, GI effects	• Risk of hypertensive crisis • Contraindicated with other serotonergic agents
Psychostimulants			
Methylphenidate Dexamphetamine Modafinil		Insomnia, agitation, tremor, anxiety, hypertension, tachycardia, arrhythmia	• Contraindicated in significant cardiovascular disease • Risk of dependence
Second-Generation Antipsychotics			
Quetiapine Olanzapine Risperidone Aripiprazole Lurasidone Asenapine	3A4 substrate 1A2 substrate 2D6 substrate 2D6 substrate 3A4 substrate 1A2 substrate	Sedation, weight gain, metabolic syndrome (diabetes, hypercholesterolemia), anticholinergic and sexual side effects	• Risk of QTc prolongation • Caution with risperidone, lurasidone, and olanzapine in breast cancer due to risk of increase in prolactin levels • May lower seizure threshold

Triiodothyronine		
T3/liothyronine		Arrhythmias, tachycardia, hypertension, headache, tremor	Contraindicated in thyrotoxicosis or adrenal insufficiency
Mood Stabilizers		
Lithium carbonate Lithium citrate	Renally cleared	Ataxia, sedation, dysarthria, delirium, tremor, cognitive dysfunction, polyuria, polydipsia, diarrhea, nausea, weight gain, thyroid toxicity, renal toxicity, acne, rash, alopecia (adverse effects are dose-related)	• Contraindicated with brain damage, renal disease (especially if low sodium diet required; absolute contraindication in severe insufficiency), cardiovascular disease and severe debilitation • Elderly have lower target serum levels
Valproate Divalproex	Moderate 2C9 and 2C19	Sedation, tremor, dizziness, ataxia, asthenia, headache, GI distress, alopecia, weight gain, impaired liver function	• Lamotrigine dose should be reduced by 50% if used with valproate • Aspirin and ibuprofen increase valproate levels • Monitor for impaired liver function • Contraindicated with thrombocytopenia ad hepatic impairment
Carbamazepine	Induces 3A4, 2C19, 2D6, 3A4 substrate	Sedation, dizziness, confusion, unsteadiness, headache, GI distress, blurred vision, rash (rarely Stevens-Johnson Syndrome), rare aplastic anemia, agranulocytosis, rarely SIADH	• Auto-induces its own metabolism • Synergistic blood dyscrasia with clozapine • Induce metabolism of oral contraceptive potentially leading to unintended pregnancy • May exacerbate angle-closure glaucoma • Must monitor for rash and blood dyscrasias

(continued)

Table 5.2 Continued

Drugs	CYP450[a]	Common Side Effects	Cautions
Lamotrigine	Metabolized by hepatic glucorunidation, not through CYP450	Sedation, blurred/double vision, dizziness, ataxia, headache, tremor, insomnia, poor coordination, fatigue, GI distress, benign rash (10%), rarely Stevens-Johnson Syndrome, rare aseptic meningitis, rare blood dyscrasias	• Lamotrigine dose should be reduced by 50% if used with valproate • Slow dose titration (6 weeks) with close monitoring to reduce risk of rash • Primarily used for bipolar depression
Benzodiazepines			
Alprazolam Clonazepam Diazepam Lorazepam Oxazepam Temazepam		Excessive sedation, dizziness, respiratory depression, paradoxical disinhibition	• Potential for addiction and tolerance • Risk of falls and cognitive impairment, particularly in elderly • May be deliriogenic • Taper slowly to avoid withdrawal and rebound anxiety
Anticonvulsants (as adjuncts for anxiety)			
Pregabalin Gabapentin		Dizziness, drowsiness, dry mouth, peripheral edema, ataxia blurred vision, weight gain, cognitive dysfunction	
β-blockers (as adjuncts for anxiety)			
Atenolol Propanalol Pindolol Clonidine (α- agonist)		Bradycardia, hypotension, bronchospasm, dizziness, vertigo	• Exacerbation of vascular disease and Raynaud's • Increases adverse effects of gabapentin and benzodiazepines

Antihistamines (off-label adjuncts for anxiety)		
Hydroxyzine Diphenhydramine Dimenhydrinate	Dry mouth, sedation, tremor; cognitive dysfunction, constipation, rare respiratory depression	• Synergistic effect with other central nervous system depressants • Enhanced anticholinergic effects
Hypnotics		
Eszopiclone Zopiclone Zaleplon Zolpidem	Headache, dry mouth, dizziness, somnolence, nausea, myalgias, rarely sleep eating syndrome or hallucinations	• Taper slowly to prevent rebound insomnia • Caution with zaleplon in hepatic or renal insufficiency
Emerging Therapies		
Nabilone/Cannabis	• Ongoing studies assessing cannabis and nabilone for anxiety and neuropathic pain	
Ketamine	• Ongoing clinical trials assessing ketamine for rapid antidepressant and anxiolytic effects	
Alternative Therapies		
St. John's Wort Omega-3 SAM-e	• May be helpful for mild to moderate depression • May be preferred by patients with cancer reluctant to consider pharmaceutical antidepressants • Lack of standardization in formulation and dose in most countries • Limited knowledge of drug interactions	

Note: QTc: corrected QT; GI: gastrointestinal; SNRI: selective norepinephrine reuptake inhibitors; NDRI: norepinephrine–dopamine reuptake inhibitor; NRI: norepinephrine reuptake inhibitor; NaSSA: noradrenergic and specific serotonergic antidepressant; SARI: serotonin antagonist and reuptake inhibitor; SPARI: serotonin partial agonist reuptake inhibitor; SMS: serotonin modulator and stimulator; SAM-e: S-adenosylmethionine; SIADH: syndrome of inappropriate antidiuretic hormone secretion.

[a] Only moderate or strong cytochrome P450 inhibition shown, or substrate status where indicated.

[b] Melatonergic agonist and serotonergic antagonist, increasing release of dopamine and norepinephrine.

Table 5.3 Commonly Prescribed Psychotropics in Cancer

Generic Name	Standard Adult Dose	Therapeutic Considerations
Antidepressants		
Citalopram/ Escitalopram	Start: 10 to 20 mg daily (od) / (5 to 10 mg qhs) Goal: 20 to 40 mg / (10 to 20 mg) Max: 40 mg od / (20 mg qhs)	• May help with hot flashes • Escitalopram may have more rapid onset than other SSRIs (1 to 3 weeks)
Venlafaxine/ Desvenlafaxine	Start: 37.5 to 75 mg qam / (50 mg) Goal: 75 to 225 mg / (50 to 100 mg) Max: 300 mg qam / (100 mg)	• Optimal choice for patients on tamoxifen • Consider for prominent hot flashes
Bupropion XL	Start: 150 mg qam Goal: 150 to 300 mg Max: 450 mg qam	• Consider for prominent fatigue • Aids sexual function • Smoking cessation aid • Weight neutral
Duloxetine	Start: 30 mg qam Goal: 30 to 60 mg Max: 120 mg qam	• Separate indications for neuropathic and chronic pain
Mirtazapine	Start: 7.5 to 15 mg po qhs Goal: 15 to 45 mg Max: 60 mg po qhs	• Consider for prominent insomnia, anorexia/cachexia, anxiety, nausea, diarrhea, pruritus • Rapid-dissolve formulation available
Select Antipsychotics[a]		
Quetiapine	Start: 25 mg qhs Goal: 100 to 400 mg qhs Max: 600 mg qhs	• May help with insomnia from depression, anxiety or steroid induced • Associated with increased appetite and significant weight gain
Olanzapine	Start: 2.5 mg qhs Goal: 5 to 15 mg qhs Max: 20 mg qhs	• May help with insomnia from depression, anxiety or steroid induced • Associated with increased appetite and significant weight gain

Risperidone	Start: 0.25 mg qhs or bid Goal: 1 to 4 mg (qhs or split into bid) Max: 6 mg (qhs or split into bid)	• Less sedating than quetiapine and olanzapine • Highest risk of extrapyramidal symptoms of all second-generation antipsychotics
Aripiprazole	Start: 2.5 mg od Goal: 2.5 to 10 mg od Max: 15 mg od	• May be activating • Associated with gastroparesis and akathisia at high doses • Weight neutral
Benzodiazepines		
Lorazepam	Dosing: 0.5 to 2 mg q4h prn Onset: Intermediate Duration: Intermediate $t_{1/2}$: 10–20 hrs	• Insomnia • Panic attacks • Anticonvulsant
Clonazepam	Dosing: 0.5 to 2 mg up to tid prn Onset: Intermediate Duration: Long $t_{1/2}$: 20–50 hrs	• Insomnia • Persistent anxiety • Anticonvulsant
Diazepam	Dosing: 2 to 60 mg od prn Onset: Fast Duration: Long $t_{1/2}$: 30–100 hrs	• Anxiety • Alcohol withdrawal • Muscle relaxant • Anticonvulsant
Alprazolam	Dosing: 0.5 to 3 mg od prn Onset: Fast Duration: Short $t_{1/2}$: 10–20 hrs	• Panic attacks • Specific phobias • Claustrophobia

Note: od: once daily; qhs: bedtime; qam: mornings; q4h: take four hourly; tid: three times a day; po: orally; prn: use when needed.
[a]Augmentation dosing for depression or anxiety.

other classes of medications, SSRIs are preferable because they have the best tolerability and the lowest risk of adverse effects and drug–drug interactions. As well, many SSRIs are now available in elixir formulations that are most convenient for those with swallowing difficulties.

Among the SSRIs, fluoxetine, paroxetine, and fluvoxamine are less desirable because of their poorer tolerability and increased propensity for drug–drug interactions via inhibition of cytochrome (CY) P450 enzymes. Citalopram and escitalopram have the best tolerability with the least drug–drug interactions. However, corrected QT (QTc) prolongation with those medications has been noted, which may of be particular concern when other QT-prolonging medications are being used. This effect is dose-dependent, with inconclusive evidence of risk in the usual dose ranges but known increased risk above maximum recommended doses. Sertraline also has good tolerability and may reduce hot flashes.

Selective norepinephrine reuptake inhibitors

The efficacy and tolerability of selective norepinephrine reuptake inhibitors (SNRIs) is comparable to the SSRIs, and they have an added potential benefit of improving neuropathic pain; therefore, SNRIs are also considered as a first-line treatment. The short-term and long-term adverse effects of SNRIs are essentially the same as SSRIs, although they may increase blood pressure at higher doses due to increased norepinephrine levels.

Venlafaxine and its metabolite desvenlafaxine are often well tolerated, with fewer CYP450 interactions, than other antidepressants. They also have very low protein binding and are therefore unlikely to displace other protein-bound medications. Further, both antidepressants are effective to treat hot flashes associated with estrogen modulators in breast cancer and with androgen ablation therapy in prostate cancer. However, venlafaxine has a short half-life, and therefore even a single missed dose may cause significant serotonin discontinuation symptoms. There is strong evidence for the benefit of duloxetine for neuropathic pain, although it has been associated with elevated serum transaminase and bilirubin levels.

Tricyclic antidepressants

The efficacy of tricyclic antidepressants (TCAs) is comparable to SSRIs, although their tolerability is much poorer. This may account for their discontinuation by up to one-third of medically ill patients prior to completion of treatment. Therefore, TCAs are generally inadvisable for the primary treatment of major depression in cancer, although they may be cautiously used in low doses for the treatment of insomnia and neuropathic pain. A trial of TCAs may be indicated when there has been inadequate antidepressant response to newer agents or when there is neuropathic pain. In such cases, newer generation TCAs (e.g., desipramine, lofepramine, and nortryptiline) should preferentially be selected, as they are associated with fewer anticholinergic and cardiotoxic effects.

Atypical antidepressants

Several antidepressant agents with alternate mechanisms of action may also be effective in the treatment of major depression in cancer. Mirtazapine may have utility when insomnia and/or cachexia are comorbid with depression because of the sedation and appetite stimulation that occurs with this medication. Mirtazapine has additional benefits of not causing adverse gastrointestinal side effects, having an antiemetic effect and being available in an orally disintegrating tablet (mirtazapine ODT) that is well tolerated by patients with difficulty swallowing.

Bupropion has simulating effects, which may be particularly helpful for patients with prominent fatigue and/or amotivation. It also has benefits of facilitating smoking cessation and in improving in sexual dysfunction, but should be avoided when there is comorbid anxiety, as it may exacerbate these symptoms. Buroproprion may also lower the seizure threshold and so should be avoided in patients with primary or secondary brain cancer or in those with a history of seizures or head injury. Of note, SSRIs should be selected for the treatment of depression of anxiety in patients with a seizure disorder and/or a cerebral tumor, as these agents have less propensity to decrease the seizure threshold.

Agomelatine, a melatonin analog, may be particularly helpful for improving sleep patterns in depressed patients. It has not yet been studied in cancer patients, and evidence for its effectiveness in depression in psychiatric populations is just emerging. However, it appears to have only mild side effects, to be relatively safe in overdose, and its discontinuation is not followed by a withdrawal syndrome.

Vortioxetine has been found to improve cognitive function, independent of its antidepressant effect, and therefore may have particular value for patients with cognitive dysfunction, although this effect has not been substantiated in clinical trials.

Atypical or second-generation antipsychotics

Second-generation antipsychotics (SGAs) are effective as augmenting agents in the treatment of major depression and anxiety disorders in the general population, although this effect has not been studied in cancer patients with these disorders. However, antipsychotics used for this purpose may have additional benefit in cancer patients by stimulating appetite, relieving chemotherapy-induced nausea, improving sleep, and alleviating perceptual disturbances associated with delirium. When there has been only a partial or incomplete response to the pharmacological treatment of depression or anxiety, particularly when symptoms of insomnia, anorexia, or nausea persist, an SGA may be added to achieve remission. Olanzapine, quetiapine, and aripiprazole have the greatest evidence to support their use as augmenting agents for depression in the general population. Olanzapine and quetiapine tend to cause sedation, weight gain, and metabolic side effects, although these effects may be advantageous for cancer patients with anorexia and insomnia. Aripiprazole is preferable when these side effects should be avoided.

Psychostimulants

Psychostimulants are frequently utilized off-label for fatigue or depression in the medically ill. Evidence of their effectiveness for depression in cancer patients is unclear and contradictory, although that for improvement of symptoms of fatigue, cognitive dysfunction, apathy, amotivation, and psychomotor retardation is stronger. Psychostimulants have a rapid onset of action, with effects observed almost immediately, and therefore may be of particular benefit in palliative care settings when life expectancy is limited. Stimulants have minimal drug–drug interactions but should be used with caution in patients with significant comorbid anxiety, dementia, anorexia, or insomnia or in the presence of cardiac disease.

Prescribing an Antidepressant for Major Depression in Cancer

Factors that should be considered when selecting among the various classes of available antidepressants are outlined in Box 5.3. The choice of medication should be tailored to the patient's depressive symptoms, the antidepressant side-effect profile, and the clinical context.

In the context of drug-induced mood episodes (e.g., steroid-related depression), removal of the offending agent and/or addition of an antidepressant are the primary pharmacologic interventionse. When the offending agent is medically necessary, the potential costs and benefits of continuing versus discontinuing it must be weighed on a case-by-case basis. In the case of steroid therapy, mood effects may persist or even be precipitated by discontinuation of this medication. If steroids must be maintained, it is often helpful to augment antidepressant medications with SGAs, particularly if insomnia is prominent. For patients who do not have a history of previous depressive episodes and if the episode is clearly drug-induced, antidepressant treatment may be stopped a few months after depressive symptoms have resolved if the drug has been discontinued.

First-line agents for the treatment of major depression include SSRIs, SNRIs, norepinephrine and dopamine reuptake inhibitors (i.e., bupropion), and noradrenergic and specific serotonergic antidepressants (i.e., mirtazapine).

Box 5.3 Considerations for Selecting an Antidepressant

- Previous responsiveness to a specific antidepressant
- Family history of responsiveness to a specific antidepressant
- Concurrent medications (i.e., potential drug–drug interactions)
- Somatic symptom profile (e.g., sedating antidepressant for those with prominent insomnia; weight-gaining antidepressant for cachectic patients)
- Potential for dual benefit (e.g., duloxetine and TCAs for neuropathic pain, venlafaxine for hot flashes)
- Type of cancer (e.g., avoid bupropion in those with central nervous system cancers)
- Comorbidities (e.g. avoid psychostimulants or TCAs with comorbid cardiac disease)
- Cancer prognosis (e.g., consider psychostimulants with very short life expectancy)

Dosing and therapeutic considerations for the most commonly prescribed antidepressants in patients with cancer are described in Table 5.3 (page 90).

For a first major depressive episode, daily antidepressant therapy at the dose required initially to achieve remission should be continued for an additional 6 to 12 months. Following recurrent major depressive episodes, a minimum of two consecutive years of treatment is indicated. If there have been four or more major depressive episodes, lifetime maintenance on antidepressants is recommended to prevent relapse.

Only two-thirds of all patients with major depression have an initial response to an antidepressant, and depressive symptoms in cancer patients may be more resistant to treatment and have a higher risk of relapse than in general psychiatric populations. Standard approaches to an inadequate response to an initial antidepressant trial include optimizing dosage, switching to another class of antidepressant, or combining antidepressant classes or augmentation, as illustrated in Figure 5.2. In rare cases, neurostimulation techniques delivered by psychiatric specialists are effective in the treatment of refractory depression.

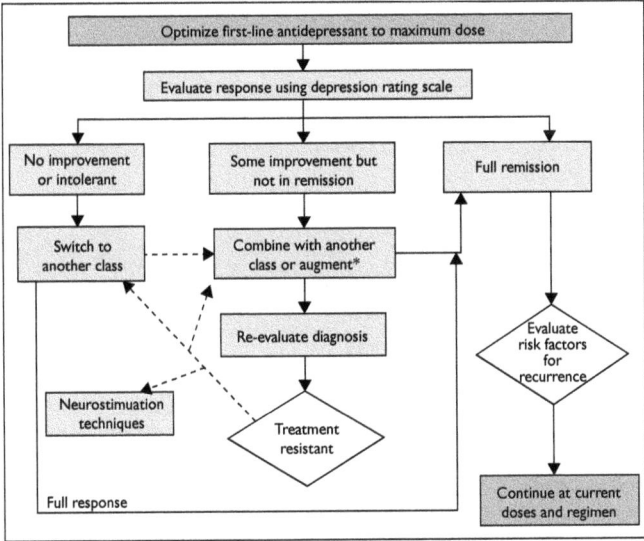

Figure 5.2. Algorithm for managing limited response to first-line treatment for depression. *Augmenting agents include lithium, triiodothyronine, atypical antipsychotics, or buspirone.

Case Study

Depression

Ms. J is a 38-year-old woman, married with children ages one and three. While still breastfeeding, she was diagnosed with stage IV breast cancer with metastases to the liver and lung. Ms. J presented with symptoms of sadness and anxiety, existential distress, and difficulty initiating sleep. She was hopeful that chemotherapy would prolong her life and her symptoms did not meet diagnostic criteria for an anxiety or mood disorder. She had no personal psychiatric history, although she reported a history of depression in her mother and brother. Ms. J developed severe hot flashes on tamoxifen and was started on venlafaxine 37.5 mg qam, with significant benefit. She and her husband actively engaged in supportive counseling focused on leaving a legacy for her children. MS J later developed brain metastases, treated initially with brain radiation and then steroids; she subsequently developed steroid-induced diabetes. Ms. J then reported significantly more insomnia, feelings of disengagement from her children, and losing interest in completing legacy projects. She was self-critical about her impatience and irritability with her family, felt persistently sad and hopeless, and had thoughts that she would be better off dead, although she denied suicidal intent. Her venlafaxine was titrated up to 150 mg, followed by significant resolution of her depressive symptoms over the following six weeks. However, as her steroids were tapered, Ms. J's depression relapsed, with worsening insomnia, anergia, and anorexia, as well as daily vomiting with meals. Her venlafaxine was initially increased to 225 mg, but this resulted in an elevation in her blood pressure with no benefit to her mood over the following three weeks. Her venlafaxine was, therefore, reduced to 150 mg and olanzapine 5 mg qhs was added and subsequently titrated to 10 mg qhs. This regimen provided significant improvement in her sleep, appetite, mood, and nausea.

Ms. J was maintained on venlafaxine 150 mg and olanzapine 10 mg qhs, and she and her husband continued in joint counseling. Although she experienced a brief upsurge in emotional distress while preparing her children for her death, she remained otherwise euthymic. Ms. J completed all of her planned legacy projects and died peacefully.

Pharmacological Management of Anxiety in Cancer

Antianxiety Medication Classes

First-line antidepressants, antipsychotics, or hypnotics may be prescribed for anxiety disorders (see chapter 2). Beta-blockers, clonidine, and antihistamines have occasionally been used as adjunctive agents for anxiety, although there is very limited evidence for their effectiveness (Table 5.2, p. 86). Beta-blockers and clonidine are also occasionally used to alleviate hot flashes and so may be appropriate when such a dual benefit of action is desired. Benzodiazepines, anticonvulsants, and buspirone have a stronger evidence base to support their use as adjunctive agents in the treatment of anxiety.

Benzodiazepines

Several considerations and cautions should be taken into account when prescribing benzodiazepines in cancer populations. Most benzodiazepines are metabolized in the liver, with the exception of lorazepam, oxazepam, and temazepam, and this may be impaired when cancer involves the liver. As well, sedation, psychomotor impairment, and dizziness are common and potentially problematic adverse effects of benzodiazepines., Benzodiazepines have occasionally been associated with ataxia, blurred vision, low blood pressure, and memory disturbance. Therefore, patients regularly using these medications should be advised to avoid driving or engaging in other activities that require close attention. Due to these adverse effects and because of the high frequency of physiological tolerance, bezodiasepines should be used only for short-term indications. These include anxiety symptoms that occur in specific situations, such as claustrophobia with medical imaging, temporary insomnia, or to abort panic attacks. The onset of action and duration of effect for benzodiazepines should be considered in their selection for specific clinical situations (see Table 5.3, p. 91).

Patients who suffer from panic attacks may use benzodiazepines as a backup plan, when breathing and relaxation strategies are not effective to alleviate occasional attacks. The mere availability of this medication available may, in itself, relieve anxiety. However, when panic symptoms are severe and persistent, despite regular daily doses of benzodiazepines, treatment with an antidepressant such as an SSRI is indicated.

Anticonvulsants (pregabalin and gabapentin)

Gabapentin and pregabalin have a modest anxiolytic effect and may also be used in the treatment of seizures, neuropathic pain, restless leg syndrome, and hot flashes. Their anxiolytic effectiveness has yet to be established in patients with cancer but they may be used as adjunctive agents when there has been only partial remission with an antidepressant. Pregabalin has been more extensively studied in the treatment of anxiety in the general population and has been recommended in the treatment of generalized anxiety disorder. Its anxiolytic effects may not appear until a few weeks after treatment initiation.

Buspirone

Buspirone is a $5\text{-}HT_{1A}$ partial agonist that has been shown to have anxiolytic and antidepressant effects in the general population, although this has not been evaluated in patients with cancer. It is primarily used as a non-benzodiazepine alternative in the treatment of generalized anxiety disorder. The onset of the anxiolytic effect of buspirone may take several weeks, but it may still be preferable to benzodiazepines because of its better tolerability and safety profile. Buspirone is associated with minimal sedation, psychomotor slowing, cognitive dysfunction, or respiratory depression and has no associated risk of addiction or tolerance.

General Principles of Pharmacologic Management of Anxiety Disorders in Cancer

Antidepressants are first line treatments for most DSM-5 defined anxiety disorders, including generalized anxiety disorder, panic disorder, social phobia, and obsessive-compulsive disorder. The same general prescribing practices that apply to first-line agents for depression also apply to the treatment of anxiety disorders. These include attention to tolerability, drug–drug interactions, and specific off-target effects for dual benefit. Of note, although bupropion and stimulants are used to treat major depression, they may actually exacerbate symptoms of anxiety.

Although not categorized as anxiety disorders in the DSM-5, adjustment disorder and posttraumatic stress disorder (PTSD) are often grouped with anxiety disorders in cancer. Due to its self-limited nature, adjustment disorder would rarely warrant pharmacotherapy, aside from short-term use of benzodiazepines or hypnotics as needed. The recommended pharmacologic treatment of PTSD is similar to the other anxiety disorders, with antidepressants as first-line treatments, and augmentation with SGAs as required.

Dosing and titration principles of antidepressants for anxiety vary somewhat from those for depression. With anxiety, dosing should start low and increase slowly because of the propensity of antidepressants to cause initial exacerbation of symptoms of anxiety (see Box 5.4). Avoiding such treatment-emergent anxiety may diminish treatment discontinuation.

Box 5.4

For anxiety, the general rule for antidepressant dosing is *start low, go slow, and aim high*.

Higher doses of antidepressants are often required to achieve full remission of anxiety, and the lag time to the onset of treatment effect is greater for anxiolytic than for the antidepressant effect. Whereas an antidepressant effect may be evident in four to six weeks, the full anxiolytic effect of these medications may require eight to twelve weeks of treatment at an adequate dose. Practitioners should be aware of this to avoid premature assumptions of treatment resistance and the need to switch to another first-line antidepressant for anxiety. A pharmacological algorithm for the treatment of anxiety in patients with cancer is shown in Figure 5.3 (page 99).

For those with severe anxiety requiring immediate relief, a benzodiazepine may be initiated along with an antidepressant, with tapering of the benzodiazepine dosage once the antidepressant has achieved a therapeutic effect. For patients who can tolerate waiting for an antidepressant to take effect, a first-line antidepressant alone may be sufficient. If no effect is obtained after an adequate trial at an adequate dose or if the antidepressant is not well tolerated, a switch to another antidepressant may be indicated. Once a response to a first-line antidepressant is observed, the dose may be optimized to maximize the anxiolytic effects. If full remission is not achieved on initial therapy, augmentation with an SGA, an anticonvulsant, or buspirone is recommended. Augmentation with these agents is preferable to long-term use of benzodiazepines due to lower risk of respiratory depression, cognitive dysfunction, and dependence. SGA augmentation has the greatest evidence for its augmentation effect, but the augmenting agent should be switched if no additional benefit is observed or if it is poorly tolerated. When full remission is achieved, the combination of medications should be continued at the same doses for at least one to two years or until the triggering stressor is no longer present.

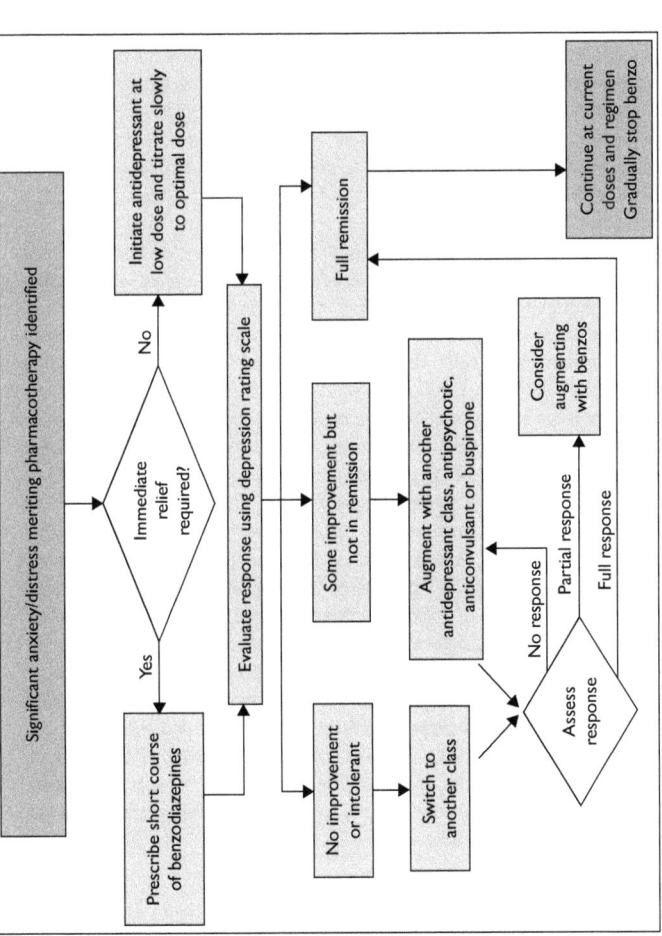

Figure 5.3. Algorithm for pharmacologic treatment of anxiety.

Case Studies

Anxiety

Case 1

Ms. S was a 64 year old artist, single, with no children who was investigated for persistent gastrointestinal symptoms and a colorectal mass identified on imaging. A biopsy was booked, but she repeatedly canceled and then rebooked appointments over a period of three months. This was related to indecision about the treatment, with long periods of time spent on the Internet searching for information about colon cancer and alternative therapies. She eventually decided that she would refuse treatment, even if she did have colon cancer, because the thought of going through surgery and chemotherapy was too overwhelming. She had no living family and was unaccustomed to turning to friends for support.

Ms. S reported symptoms of anxiety that were constant and all-consuming and associated with insomnia and diffuse body pain that interfered with painting, which she engaged in to distract herself from her worry. She was often nauseous and unable to eat and had lost 15 pounds. Although she had never sought treatment for anxiety in the past, Ms. S described herself as have always been "a worrier" such that "if you tell me 90% equals good chances, and 10% bad—the 10% weighs a ton in my mind." She had avoided medical check-ups and colonoscopy screening, despite chronic worry about developing cancer, and had always preferred natural approaches to treatment, as she feared medication side effects.

Ms. S was referred for psychiatric assessment and intervention. The initial focus was on developing a therapeutic alliance, exploring her need for control to regulate anxiety, and helping her to engage her social support network. She eventually agreed to take lorazepam 2 mg at home to allow her to come to her biopsy appointment. A diagnosis of colorectal adenocarcinoma with liver metastases was made on biopsy, and she agreed to undergo surgery and receive chemotherapy. Ms. S was maintained on clonazepam 2 mg at bedtime for sleep at her request until after her surgery. After the first month of chemotherapy, she developed panic attacks triggered by the thought of coming to treatment, and she missed two scheduled chemotherapy dates. She was subsequently started on escitalopram, titrated to 20 mg daily, with good response. Ms. S was then able to complete six months of chemotherapy and was maintained on escitalopram, with eventual weaning off of her clonazepam.

Case 2

Mr. B was a 49 year-old man, divorced, with two teenage children, and working as a civil engineer. He was found to have an adenocarcinoma in his cervical lymph nodes, presumed to be metastatic, although a primary tumor site was not confirmed. He was scheduled to begin a five-week course of radiotherapy but was struggling with significant anxiety about being immobilized under a radiation mask. His past medical history was significant for chronic obstructive pulmonary disease, with a 30-pack/year history of smoking, and regular use *of a roflumilast inhaler. Mr. B had a long history of claustrophobia, marked by anxiety on crowded elevators, traveling on subway cars during rush hour, and flying on airplanes. He had avoided these situations throughout his life and had never previously sought treatment for his anxiety symptoms. He prepared for treatment by learning progressive muscle relaxation techniques and by bringing music to the treatment sessions to distract himself but nevertheless experienced a severe panic attack during radiation planning. He feared that taking medications for anxiety that caused sedation would prevent him from returning to work after his daily radiation treatment was completed. Therefore, Mr. B was prescribed alprazolam, based on its properties of rapid onset and short duration, 1 mg to be taken one hour prior to each radiation treatment, combined with his music and relaxation exercises. With this regimen, he was able to complete radiation treatment successfully and to participate in graduated exposure therapy to address his claustrophobia more definitively.*

Drug Interactions

Many reliable drug interaction checkers are now readily available through free or institutional programs such as Lexicomp, Epocrates, Medscape, or RxList. Table 5.4 also lists specific drug interactions of concern between oncology medications and psychotropics. Many common antineoplastic agents have no significant pharmacokinetic drug interactions with antidepressants, including temozolomide, 5-fluorouracil, gemcitabine, platinum-based chemotherapy, or anthracycline agents. Antidepressants with the least impact on CYP450 enzymes are generally the safest options with antineoplastic agents (see Box 5.5), although these medications and, in fact, most psychotropics, have been associated with prolonged QTc intervals. Physicians are encouraged to consult the Arizona Center for Education and Research on Therapeutics for regularly updated information on QT drug lists (http://www.QTdrugs.org).

When prescribing SSRIs, it is important to monitor for serotonin syndrome. Serotonin syndrome is a rare occurrence, observed mainly when multiple serotonergic agents are combined (e.g., St. John's Wort and an SSRI, SNRI plus SSRI). This potentially lethal syndrome is characterized by a clinical triad of cognitive effects (headache, agitation, hypomania, mental confusion, hallucinations, coma), autonomic effects (shivering, sweating, hyperthermia, vasoconstriction, tachycardia, nausea, diarrhea), and somatic effects (myoclonus, hyperreflexia, tremor). Patients should be educated about these signs and symptoms and told to immediately discontinue antidepressants and seek urgent medical attention if they are experiencing this triad.

Psychotropic drug interactions are also important considerations when managing cancer patients with delirium. Antidepressant agents

Table 5.4 Psychotropic-Oncology Drug Interactions

Oncology Drug	Psychotropics	Comments
Tamoxifen	Avoid paroxetine, fluoxetine, high-dose sertraline, bupropion	Conversion to active metabolite endoxifen reduced by potent CYP 2D6 inhibitors
Abiraterone	Avoid TCAs, aripiprazole Caution with fluoxetine, fluvoxamine, paroxetine, sertraline	May increase levels by CYP 2D6 and 2C8 inhibition
All cytotoxic agents	Avoid mianserin	Risk of bone marrow suppression
PKIs (e.g., imatinib, nilotinib, sorafenib, sunitinib, trastuzumab)	Avoid TCAs due to QTc prolongation	Nilotinib inhibits CYP 3A4 and 2D6; caution with all antidepressants
Cyclophosphamide, procarbazine, dacarbazine	Caution with paroxetine, fluoxetine, sertraline, fluvoxamine, bupropion	Effectiveness reduced by CYP 2B6, 2C19, and 1A inhibitors
Alkylating agents (ifosfamide, thiotepa)	Caution with fluoxetine, sertraline, paroxetine, fluvoxamine	Effectiveness reduced by CYP 3A4 inhibitors
Corticosteroids, etoposide, PKIs, antimicrotubules (paclitaxel, docetaxel, vinblastine, vincristine)	Caution with fluoxetine, sertraline, paroxetine, fluvoxamine	Increased levels and toxicity by CYP 3A4 inhibitors
Irinotecan	Avoid SSRIs	Risk of rhabdomyolysis and severe diarrhea
Posaconazole	Caution with quetiapine	Combination increases quetiapine levels and risk of QTc prolongation
Arsenic	Caution with all antidepressants and antipsychotics	Combination increases risk of QTc prolongation

Note: TCAs: tricyclic antidepressants; PKIs: protein kinase inhibitors; SSRIs: selective serotonin reuptake inhibitors.

with significant anticholinergic properties (i.e., mirtazapine, paroxetine, TCAs) should be discontinued or held, and potentially deliriogenic agents (i.e., benzodiazepines, antihistamines, narcotics) should be used with caution.

Box 5.5

In general, citalopram/escitalopram, venlafaxine/desvenlafaxine, and mirtazapine are antidepressant options with the fewest drug interactions.

Service Implementation

Pharmacotherapy should generally be reserved for more severe anxiety and depressive presentations and may be most effective when combined with psychotherapeutic interventions. Notably, pharmacotherapy may also be considered for mild to moderate symptoms that are persistent or that interfere with engagement in cancer treatment. The stepped care model from the National Institute for Health and Care Excellence provides clear guidance on these intervention options, based on depression severity, duration, and course (https://www.nice.org.uk/guidance/cg91/chapter/1-Guidance#stepped-care).[12] Adapted for anxiety and depression in cancer, this model suggests provision of basic support and psychoeducation to all cancer patients and delivery of lower intensity psychological interventions for persistent mild symptoms or subthreshold disorders, followed by progression to higher intensity interventions for persistent subthreshold or severe symptoms (Figure 5.4).[12]

Stepped care is integral to the new collaborative care models of care delivery, which are emerging as a highly effective systems-level intervention for depression in cancer. Collaborative care models are comprised of systematic case finding through screening and integrated delivery of care, achieved by active collaboration among oncologists, patient care managers, and consulting psychiatrists as needed. Care managers may provide low-intensity interventions, such as problem-solving therapy, and monitor progress with rating scales so that the intensity of intervention can be adjusted as needed. Such an approach fosters coordination of care between the oncology team and psychosocial specialists, thereby improving access to mental health services for cancer patients. Collaborative care interventions combine treatment modalities and result in more effective dose titration of medications and stronger and longer term depression remissions than obtained with pharmacotherapy or psychotherapy alone.[7] Details regarding implementation of a collaborative care model of service delivery can be obtained at http://www.teamcarehealth.org/ or http://impact-uw.org/.

Conclusion

Depression and anxiety are common symptoms in cancer patients that may adversely affect subjective well-being and quality of life and may increase the risk of treatment noncompliance and suicide. Psychotherapeutic interventions are effective in most cases of mild to moderate symptoms. More severe or persistent symptoms of anxiety or depression may benefit from treatment with antidepressant medication, combined with psychotherapeutic approaches. SSRIs are the most commonly used medications for this purpose, although a variety of other medications are also available. The choice of medications in this circumstance is typically based on the optimal side-effect profile and on other desired therapeutic effects. Timely and effective treatment of anxiety and depression may significantly enhance quality of life in cancer patients, facilitate the effective conduct of cancer treatment, support the return to premorbid levels of functioning for those with curative disease, and reduce or prevent symptoms for those with advanced or progressive disease.

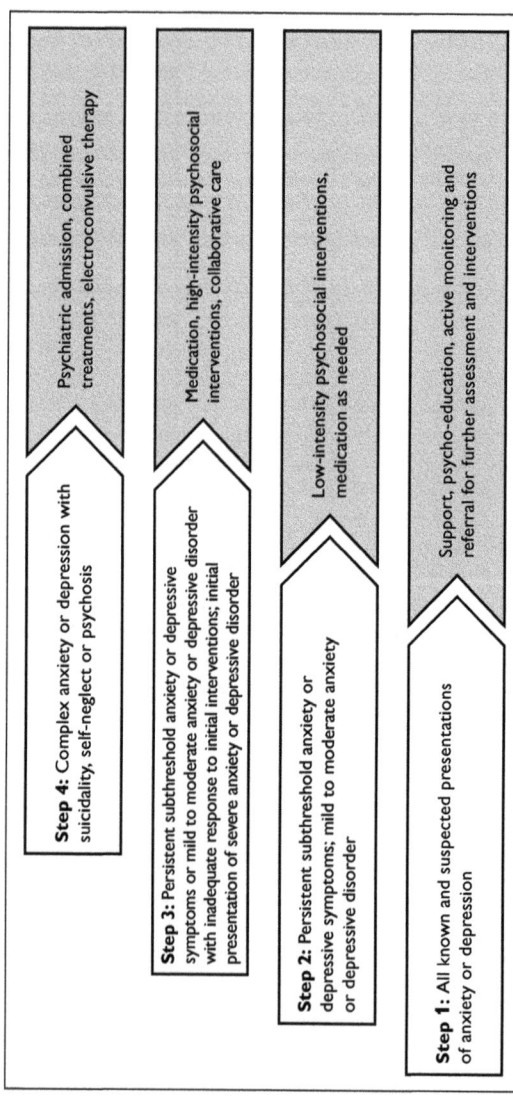

Figure 5.4. Stepped care model. Low-intensity psychosocial interventions: structured group physical activity programs, group-based peer support or self-help programs, guided self-help programs based on cognitive behavioral therapy (CBT), behavioral activation, or problem-solving techniques. High-intensity psychosocial interventions: individual or group CBT, behavioral couples' therapy, individual or group supportive-expressive psychotherapies.

References

1. Mitchell AJ, Chan M, Bhatti H, et al. Prevalence of depression, anxiety, and adjustment disorder in oncological, haematological, and palliative-care settings: a meta-analysis of 94 interview-based studies. *Lancet Oncol.* 2011;12(2):160–174.

2. Li M, Boquiren V, Lo C, et al. Depression and anxiety in supportive oncology. In: Davis M, Feyer P, Ortner P, et al., eds. *Supportive Oncology.* 1st ed. Philadelphia, PA: Elsevier; 2011:528–540.

3. Kangas M, Henry JL, Bryant RA. The course of psychological disorders in the 1st year after cancer diagnosis. *J Consult Clin Psychol.* 2005;73:763–768.

4. American Psychiatric Association. *Diagnostic and Statistical Manual of Mental Disorders.* 5th ed. Arlington, VA, American Psychiatric Association; 2013.

5. Hegerl U, Schonknecht P, Mergl R. Are antidepressants useful in the treatment of minor depression? a critical update of the current literature. *Curr Opin Psychiatry.* 2012;25(1):1–6.

6. Li M, Fitzgerald P, Rodin G. Evidence-based treatment of depression in patients with cancer. *J Clin Oncol.* 2012;30(11):1187–1196.

7. Li, M, Kennedy EB, Byrne N, et al. The management of depression in patients with cancer: a quality initiative of the Program in Evidence-Based Care (PEBC), Cancer Care Ontario (CCO). Guideline #19-4. Toronto: Cancer Care Ontario; May 2015.

8. Traeger, Greer JA, Fernandez-Robles C, et al. Evidence-based treatment of anxiety in patients with cancer. *J Clin Oncol.* 2012;30(11):1197–1205.

9. Katzman MA, Bleau P, Blier P, et al. Canadian clinical practice guidelines for the management of anxiety, posttraumatic stress and obsessive-compulsive disorders. *BMC Psychiatry.* 2014;14(Suppl 1):S1.

10. Ramasubbu R, Taylor VH, Samaan Z, et al. The Canadian Network for Mood and Anxiety Treatments (CANMAT) Task Force recommendations for the management of patients with mood disorders and select comorbid medical conditions. *Ann Clin Psychiatry.* 2012;24(1):91–109.

11. Lo C, Zimmermann C, Rydall A, et al. Longitudinal study of depressive symptoms inpatients with metastatic gastrointestinal and lung cancer. *J Clin Oncol.* 2010;28(18):3084–3089.

12. National Institute for Health and Care Excellence. Depression in adults: the treatment and management of depression in adults. NICE Clinical Guideline 90. London: British Psychological Society and Royal College of Psychiatrists; 2010. https://www.nice.org.uk/guidance/cg91/evidence/full-guideline-243876061

Further Reading

Caruso R, Grassi L, Nanni MG, Riba M. Psychopharmacology in psycho-oncology. *Curr Psychiatry Rep.* 2013 Sep;15(9):393.

Grassi L, Caruso R, Hammelef K, Nanni MG, Riba M. Efficacy and safety of pharmacotherapy in cancer-related psychiatric disorders across the trajectory of cancer care: a review. *Int Rev Psychiatry.* 2014 Feb;26(1):44–62.

Publications that provide detailed information on prescribing psychotropics within cancer care.

Howell D, Keshavarz H, Esplen MJ, et al. *A Pan Canadian Practice Guideline: Screening, Assessment and Care of Psychosocial Distress, Depression, and Anxiety in Adults with Cancer.* Toronto: Canadian Partnership Against Cancer and the Canadian Association of Psychosocial Oncology; July 2015.

A symptom management guideline on screening, triage algorithms for assessment, and high-level treatment overview for anxiety and depression in cancer patients.

Miguel C, Albuquerque E. Drug interaction in psycho-oncology: antidepressants and antineoplastics. *Pharmacology.* 2011;88(5–6):333–339.

Comprehensive review of CYP450 drug interactions between antidepressants and antineoplastic agents.

Ostuzzi, G, Benda L, Costa E, Barbui C. Efficacy and acceptability of antidepressants on the continuum of depressive experiences in patients with cancer: systematic review and meta-analysis. *Cancer Treat Rev.* 2015;41(8):714–724.

Systematic review of antidepressants for depression (including major depression, adjustment disorder, dysthymia, or depressive symptomss) in cancer patients, current to February 2015, demonstrating positive benefit of antidepressants, positively associated with duration of treatment.

Walker J, Hansen CH, Martin P, et al. Integrated collaborative care for major depression comorbid with a poor prognosis cancer (SMaRT Oncology-3): a multicentre randomised controlled trial in patients with lung cancer. *Lancet Oncol.* 2014;15(10):1168–1176.

Third of the SmaRT (Symptom Management Research Trials) oncology randomized controlled trials demonstrating strong effectiveness of collaborative care inteventions for depression in cancer (advanced lung; OR 5.88).

Chapter Quiz

Questions

1. Pharmacotherapy for depression should be used when
   A. depression is severe.
   B. the patient has a preference for pharmacologic approaches.
   C. psychological interventions alone have been ineffective.
   D. all of the above.

2. Which statement is true regarding pharmacotherapy and psychotherapy for anxiety or depression?
   A. Pharmacotherapy is always more effective than psychotherapy.
   B. Pharmacotherapy and psychotherapy should never be combined as they are equally effective and it would be a waste of resources.
   C. Pharmacotherapy is more effective for more severe symptomatology.
   D. They should always be combined for all patients.

3. Which benzodiazepine should be avoided in patients with hepatic impairment?
   A. Clonazepam
   B. Lorazepam
   C. Oxazepam
   D. Temazepam
4. Which antidepressant dual benefit statement is false?
   A. Venlafaxine can also reduce hot flashes.
   B. Bupropion may increase energy and libido.
   C. Duloxetine is also indicated for neuropathic pain.
   D. Mirtazapine reduces hypersomnolence and weight gain.
5. Which antidepressant has the least potential for CYP450 drug interactions?
   A. Paroxetine
   B. Citalopram
   C. Duloxetine
   D. Bupropion

Appendix 1

NCCN Distress Thermometer and Problem List

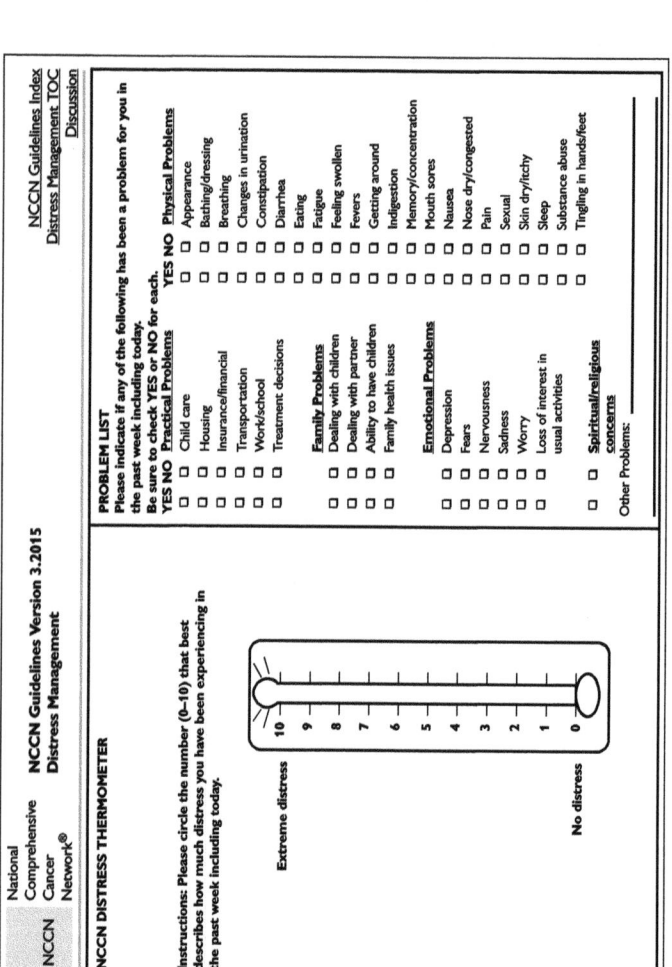

Appendix 1
National Comprehensive Cancer Network Distress Thermometer and Problem List. Adapted with permission from NCCN Guidelines

Appendix 2

Demoralization Scale-II

*For each statement below, please indicate how much (or how strongly) you have felt this way **over the last two weeks** by circling the corresponding number.*

		Never	Sometimes	Often
1	There is little value in what I can offer others.	0	1	2
2	My life seems to be pointless.	0	1	2
3	My role in life has been lost.	0	1	2
4	I no longer feel emotionally in control.	0	1	2
5	No one can help me.	0	1	2
6	I feel that I cannot help myself.	0	1	2
7	I feel hopeless.	0	1	2
8	I feel irritable.	0	1	2
9	I do not cope well with life.	0	1	2
10	I have a lot of regret about my life.	0	1	2
11	I tend to feel hurt easily.	0	1	2
12	I feel distressed about what is happening to me.	0	1	2
13	I am not a worthwhile person.	0	1	2
14	I would rather not be alive.	0	1	2
15	I feel quite isolated or alone.	0	1	2
16	I feel trapped by what is happening to me.	0	1	2

Scoring Instructions: Total score demoralization: Sum all 16 items. Scores ≥8 are of concern clinically.

Meaning and Purpose subscale: Sum items 1, 2, 3, 5, 6, 7, 13, and 14.

Distress and Coping Ability subscale: Sum items 4, 8, 9, 10, 11, 12, 15, and 16.

Reproduced with permission from *Cancer*. Robinson S, Kissane DW, Brooker J, et al. Refinement and revalidation of the Demoralization Scale: The DS-II—internal validity. *Cancer*. 2016;122(14):2251–2259; Robinson S, Kissane DW, Brooker J, et al. Refinement and revalidation of the Demoralization Scale: DS-II—external validity. *Cancer*. 2016;122(14):2260–2667.

Appendix 3

Brief Screening Tools

Beck Depression Inventory (BDI)
http://www.ibogaine.desk.nl/graphics/3639b1c_23.pdf

Distress Thermometer (DT)
http://www.nccn.org/patients/resources/life_with_cancer/pdf/nccn_distress_thermometer.pdf

Hospital Anxiety and Depression Scale (HADS)
http://www.scalesandmeasures.net/files/files/HADS.pdf

Patient Health Questionnaire (PHQ-9)
http://www.cqaimh.org/pdf/tool_phq9.pdf
This tool uses *Diagnostic and Statistical Manual of Mental Disorders* diagnostic criteria. Scores ≥10 are consistent with the diagnosis of major depressive episode.

Appendix 4

Tools for the Assessment of Suicide Risk

SAFE-T (Suicide Assessment Five-Step Evaluation and Triage)
Developed in collaboration with the Suicide Prevention Resource Center and Screening for Mental Health. (http://www.integration.samhsa.gov/images/res/SAFE_T.pdf)

Suicide Behaviors Questionnaire-Revised (SBQ-R)
Four items assessing lifetime suicide ideation and/or suicide attempt; the frequency of suicidal ideation over the past year; the threat of suicide attempt; and self-reported likelihood of suicidal behavior in the future. (http://www.integration.samhsa.gov/images/res/SBQ.pdf)

Columbia-Suicide Severity Rating Scale (C-SSRS)
Questionnaire used for suicide assessment, available in 114 country-specific languages. Various professionals can administer this scale, including physicians, nurses, psychologists, social workers, peer counselors, coordinators, research assistants, high school students, teachers, and clergy. http://www.integration.samhsa.gov/clinical-practice/Columbia_Suicide_Severity_Rating_Scale.pdf

Suicidal Ideation and Risk Level Assessment
The clinician asks suicide screening questions, determines risk factors for suicide, and then assesses suicide risk and action plan. Also the clinician asks questions that may elicit specific information relating to suicidal thoughts, plans and behaviors. http://www.cqaimh.org/pdf/tool_suicide_risklevl.pdf

Appendix 5

Answers to Chapter Quizzes

Chapter 1

1. B: False-distress is not a diagnosis. It is a non-stigmatizing, agreed-upon term that is used to identify patients who may be at increased psychological risk during cancer treatment.
2. B, C, and E: DSM-5 adjustment disorders include those with anxiety, with depressed mood, and with mixed anxiety and depressed mood.
3. B: False-there is a mild or modest association. Other predisposing factors are more important (history of pre-morbid anxiety, gender, stage of disease, social situation, co-morbid medical conditions like untreated pain).
4. B: False-must be diagnosed within 3 months of the identified stressor.
5. F: Anxiety Due to General Medical Condition is the most common anxiety disorder in patients with cancer. Adjustment disorder with anxiety does not fall under the formal anxiety disorders. All others are similarly prevalent in the general population.

Chapter 2

1. D: All of the above.
2. D: All of the above.
3. E: All of the above.
4. D: Some of the psychotherapies can be provided by professionals who are not specialized in mental health, if they receive a certain amount of training.

Chapter 3

1. E: Where Tony displays helplessness, pointlessness (futility), and distress and suicidal thinking, without the development of anhedonia signifying depression.
2. C: Where Tony could be helped to focus on alternative sources of meaning beyond his work, rebuilding his morale and attending to life in the present.

Chapter 4

1. C: About 1.5 times higher than that of the general population.
2. C: Ask what the patient would do, when and how [in order to ascertain the seriousness of the suicidal intention].
3. C: See the patient as a priority, treating this as an emergency, and assess whether she is depressed.
4. E: All of the above.

Chapter 5

1. D: All of the above.
2. C: Pharmacotherapy is more effective for more severe symptomatology.
3. A: Clonazepam.
4. D: Mirtazapine reduces hypersomnolence and weight gain.
5. B: Citalopram.

Index

Note: Page numbers followed by b, f, or t, indicate a box, figure, or table, respectively

adjustment disorders, 8–13
  assessment for, 5
  case study, 13
  clinical perspective, 9
  with demoralization, 44, 45t, 48, 53f, 58
  with demoralization, case study, 48–49
  demoralization with, 48
  depression and, 26
  description, 2
  diagnostic criteria, 8–9
  differential diagnosis, 9, 26, 43, 52
  DSM-5 classification of, 2
  key symptoms and signs, 9
  management algorithm, 21f
  psychopharmacologic options, 11–13, 99
  psychotherapeutic options, 9–11
  screening advances, 22
advance directives, 68b, 75
agomelatine (melatonin analog[b]), 86t
agoraphobia, 16t
akathisia, 12b, 18, 92t
albuterol inhaler, 15
all-or-none thinking, 36t
alprazolam, 12, 19, 70, 89t, 92t
amitriptyline, 87t
antianxiety medications. See anticonvulsants; benzodiazepines; buspirone
anticholinergics
  for anxiety disorders, 17t
  cautions, 89t
  for depression, 87t
  exacerbation of anxiety from, 15, 18
  side effects, 34, 87t, 93

anticonvulsants. See also gabapentin; pregabalin
  as adjuncts, for anxiety, 89t, 97, 99, 100f
  for depression, 89t
  side effects, cautions, 89t
  for suicide ideation, 69
antidepressants. See also selective serotonin reuptake inhibitors; serotonin-norepinephrine reuptake inhibitors; tricyclic antidepressants; specific antidepressants
  for adjustment disorders, 11, 12
  for anxiety disorders, 98–99, 99b
  for depression, 31, 33, 81, 83–85, 86t–87t, 90t, 91t, 93–99
  discontinuation syndromes, 84b
  dosage determination, 12–13
  drug interactions, 102
  for generalized anxiety disorder, 19
  practical tools for prescribing, 83b–84b
  prescription factors, 95–96
  selection considerations, 95b
  side effects, 33
  for suicide risk, 68
antidepressants, atypical, 11, 86t–87t, 93–94. See also agomelatine; bupropion; mirtazapine; vortioxetine

antiemetics, 17t, 18, 33, 94
antihistamines, 89t, 97, 103
antineoplastic agents, 102
antipsychotics. See also aripiprazole; olanzapine; quetiapine; risperidone
  for adjustment disorders, 11
  for anxiety disorders, 17t, 18–19, 97, 100f
  atypical, 96f
  cautions, 18, 33, 69b, 103t
  efficacy/safety for suicide risk, 69b
  for insomnia, 85
  second-generation (SGAs), 87t, 94
  for suicide ideation, 69, 73
anxiety disorder due to another medical condition, 17t
anxiety disorders
  case studies, 19–20, 101–102
  clinical perspective, 15
  cognitive reframing for, 36–37
  complicating issues, 4b
  description, 2–3, 13
  diagnostic criteria, 14–15
  differential diagnosis, 15, 18
  DSM-5 classification, 10f, 16t–17t, 80t, 81, 98
  impact on patients, 3
  management algorithm, 10f, 32f, 82f
  physical symptoms, 4
  professional issues, service implementation, 20

INDEX

anxiety disorders (*Cont.*)
  psychopharmacologic options, 18–19, 86t–92t, 97–102
  psychotherapeutic options, 18, 81
  signs and symptoms, 14, 14t
  situational vs. debilitating, 2
  specific disorders, 15, 16t–17t, 19
anxiolytics. *See also* alprazolam; benzodiazepines
  for adjustment disorders, 11, 12
  for anxiety disorders, 19
  for depression, 31, 33
  side effects, 34
aripiprazole, 33, 87t, 92t, 94
asenapine, 87t
atenolol, 89t

Beck Depression Inventory (BDI) (BDI-II, BDI-Short Form), 27, 111
behavioral activation, 28, 35t, 37, 105f
benzodiazepines
  for adjustment disorders, 11, 12, 99
  for anxiety, 19, 89t, 97, 100f
  cautions, 97–98, 103
  for depression, 31, 33, 89t
  for insomnia in anxiety, depression, 85
  side effects, 19, 34
  for suicidal ideation, 69, 84b
  withdrawal issues, 18
benztropine, 18
β-blockers, 89t, 97
bipolar disorders, 62, 68, 89t
bupropion
  for anxiety, 86t
  cautions, 95b, 99, 103t
  for depression, 86t, 94, 95
  side effects, 34
buspirone (5-HT$_{1A}$ agonist), 87t, 96f, 98, 99, 100f

CALM (Managing Cancer and Living Meaningfully) therapy, 35t, 36, 38, 56
cannabis 90t
Cancer Care for the Whole Patient: Meeting Psychosocial Health Needs (IOM; 2008), 2
carbamazepine, 88t
case studies
  adjustment disorder, 13
  anxiety disorders, 19–20, 101–102
  demoralization, 48–52
  demoralization with adjustment disorder, 48–49
  demoralization with major depression, 49–50
  depression, 28–29, 70, 96–97
  distress management, 8
  major depression with melancholia, 51–52
  suicide risk, 70
citalopram, 86t, 91t, 93, 103b
claustrophobia, 15, 92t, 98, 102
clonazepam, 89t
clonidine (α-agonist), 89t, 97
cognitive behavioral therapy (CBT). *See also* behavioral activation
  for adjustment disorders, 10
  for anxiety, 18, 105f
  for depression, 35, 36–37, 40, 105f
  description, 35t
  for moderate demoralization, 54
  for suicide ideation, 69
cognitive biases, 36–37
cognitive-existential with meaning-centered therapy, 54–56, 55b–56b
cognitive reframing, 36–37
cognitive therapy, 36, 57

Columbia-Suicide Severity Rating Scale (C-SSRS), 112
coping. *See also* demoralization
  in adjustment disorders, 8, 9–10, 13
  anxiety and, 18
  assessment tools, 52
  in demoralization, 43, 44, 45, 45t, 47, 49, 50, 53, 57, 58
  emotion-/problem-/meaning-based, 43
  impact of poor coping, 3, 4, 8
  psychotherapeutic treatments, 37, 38
  stigma associated with, 4
corticosteroids, 12b, 15, 17t, 103t
couple therapy, 38
cyclosporine, 15

demoralization, 43–59
  with adjustment disorder, 44, 45t, 48–49, 53f, 58
  assessment of severity, 52
  background evidence, 43–44
  case studies, 48–52
  causes of, 43
  clinical management, 53–58, 53f
  coping and, 43, 44, 45, 47, 49, 50, 53, 57, 58
  diagnostic criteria, 45b, 47
  differential diagnosis, 52
  dimensional nature of, 45t
  existentially-oriented approaches, 43, 54–55
  historical background, 43–44
  key symptoms, signs, 45
  with major depression, 49–50, 51–52
  with major depression with melancholia, 51–52
  melancholia vs., 50–51
  mild demoralization, 53–54
  misdiagnosis factors, 47

moderate
    demoralization, 54–57
presenting problems,
    44–45
professional
    issues, service
        implementation, 59
psychotherapeutic
    options, 44, 49, 50,
    52, 53–58
risk factors, 46–47
severe demoralization,
    57–58
suicide ideation and, 44
vulnerability factors,
    46–47, 46t–48t
Demoralization Scale (DS),
    44, 52
Demoralization Scale-II
    (DS-II), 52, 110
depression, 24–40
    anxiety and, 18
    assessment, 30–31
    background evidence,
        24–25
    case studies, 28–29,
        96–97
    clinical interview for,
        26–27
    coping comorbidity, 3
    crying in, 9
    demoralization with,
        49–50, 51–52
    diagnostic criteria, 25b,
        26–28
    differential diagnosis, 9,
        26, 29–30
    distress and, 4, 5b
    DSM-5 categories, 80t
    dysthymia (chronic
        depression), 26, 47t
    ECT for, 34
    essential tests, 30
    HADS screening of, 5
    key symptoms, signs,
        25, 25b
    light therapy for, 34
    management algorithm,
        32f, 82f
    melancholia with, 51–52
    misdiagnosis/
        inappropriate care
        for, 28
    monitoring progress, 28
    prevalence in cancer
        patients, 24

professional
    issues, service
        implementation,
        39–40
psychopharmacologic
    options, 31, 33–35,
    85, 86t–92t, 93–97
psychotherapeutic
    options, 31, 35–39
risk factors for, 26
routine screening in,
    30–31
self-administered
    assessment, 27
severe, impact on mental
    capacity, 39
suicide ideation and, 62,
    64, 70
term clarification, 39
underrecognition,
    undertreatment of, 25
desipramine 87t
desvenlafaxine, 86t, 91t
dexamphetamine, 87t
Diagnostic and Statistical
    Manual of Mental
    Disorders (DSM), 2
Diagnostic and Statistical
    Manual of Mental
    Disorders, fifth edition
    (DSM-5)
    adjustment disorders,
        10f
    anxiety disorders, 10f,
        16t–17t, 80t, 81, 98
    depressive disorders, 80t
diazepam, 19, 89t
differential diagnosis
    for adjustment disorders,
        2, 9
    for anxiety disorders,
        15, 18
    for demoralization, 52
    for depression, 9, 26,
        29–30
    for suicide risk, 66
dignity therapy, 35t, 36, 38
dimenhydrinate, 89t
diphenhydramine, 18, 89t
distress
    in adjustment
        disorders, 26
    in anxiety disorders,
        79, 81
    assessment of, 4–7, 9,
        18, 52, 70

case study,
    management of, 8
complicating issues, 4b
in demoralization, 44,
    45t, 47t, 58, 110t
in depression, 44, 79
diagnostic features, 80t
management algorithm,
    10f, 32f
need for
    recognizing, 3, 8
nonspecific, 7–8, 45b
psychiatric workup for,
    6–7, 6b, 7b
psychological
    features, 80t
psychopharmacologic
    options, 31, 58
psychotherapeutic
    options, 37, 38
stigma and masked
    distress, 4
in suicide ideation, 44
vulnerability factors,
    5, 6b
Distress and Coping Ability
    subscale, 52
Distress Management
    Guidelines for Trauma
    and Related Stressors
    (NCCN), 10f
Distress Thermometer
    and Problem List
    (DT&PL), 2, 4, 5, 7,
    70, 109, 111
divalproex, 88t
drug interactions, 102–103,
    103t
    antidepressants, 12, 95b,
        102–103
    antipsychotics, 85
    benzodiazepines, 19
    hypnotic agents, 72b, 76f
    programs for
        checking, 102
    SAM-e, 90t
    SSRIs, 93
    stimulants, 95
    St. John's Wort, 90t
    suicide risk patients,
        72b, 76f
duloxetine, 19, 86t, 91t,
    93, 95b
dysthymia
    (chronic depression),
    26, 47t

Edmonton Symptom Assessment Scale, 31
electroconvulsive therapy (ECT), 34
emotional reasoning, 36t
Engel, G., 44
Epocrates, drug interaction checker, 102
escitalopram, 86t, 91t
 for adjustment disorder, 13
 for anxiety, 19, 86t, 101
 for depression, 86t
 drug interactions, 93, 103
eszopiclone, 90t
ethical dilemmas
 with demoralized patients, 59
 with depressed patients, 39
 with suicidal patients, 74–75
 wtih anxious patients, 20
existentially-oriented therapies, 43, 54–55
Existential Psychotherapy (Yalom), 55

family therapy
 for demoralization, 56–57
 for depression, 38–39
 for grief, 11b
Fang, C. K., 44
fluoxetine
 for anxiety, 19, 86t
 for comorbid panic disorder, 19
 for depression, 86t
 drug interactions, 93, 103t
 switching to, 84
fluvoxamine, 86t, 93, 103t
Frank, J., 44
Frankl, V., 44

gabapentin, 69, 89t, 98
generalized anxiety disorder, 3, 14
 in chronic worriers, 15
 DSM-5 diagnostic features, 16t
 psychopharmacologic options, 17–18, 19, 98
 psychotherapeutic options, 19

Generalized Anxiety Disorder, 7-item scale (GAD 7), 18
"given up–giving up" syndrome. *See* demoralization
Gruenberg, E., 44
guided therapy, 11b

haloperidol, 18
Handbook of Psychotherapy in Cancer Care (Watson and Kissane), 11b, 69
Hospital Anxiety and Depression Scale (HADS), self-report scale, 9, 18, 27, 40, 111
hydroxyzine, 89t
hypnotics. *See also* zaleplon; zolpidem
 for adjustment disorders, 11, 13
 for anxiety disorders, 18, 19, 90t, 97, 99
 for depression, 33, 90t
 for insomnia, 19, 33, 85
 for short-term insomnia, 19
 side effects, 90t

imipramine, 19, 87t
International Psycho-Oncology Society (IPOS), 2, 11b
International Union Against Cancer, 2
interpersonal psychotherapy (IPT), 35t, 37–38
item response theory modeling, 52

ketamine, 90t

labeling, 36t
lamotrigine, 88t, 89t
Lexicomp, drug interaction checker, 102
light therapy, 34
lithium, 68, 88t, 96f
lofepramine, 87t, 93
lorazepam
 for adjustment disorders, 12, 89t
 for anxiety, 89t, 101

 cautions, 19, 97
 for depression, 31, 89t
lurasidone, 87t

magnification/minimization, 36t
masked distress, 4
MD Anderson Symptom Inventory, 31
Meaning and Purpose subscale, 52
meaning-centered therapies, 11b, 38, 54–55, 55b–56b
Medscape, drug interaction checker, 102
melancholia
 demoralization vs., 50–51
 major depression with, 51–52
Memorial Symptom Assessment Scale, 52
methylphenidate dexamphetamine, 87t
metoclopramide, 18
milnacipran, 86t
mind-body approaches, 18
 for anxiety disorders, 18
mindfulness therapies, 11b, 35t, 36
mind-reading, 36t
mirtazapine
 cautions, 103
 for depression, 28, 86t, 95–96
 for insomnia, 85, 93–94
 side effects, 34
 for suicide ideation, 68
mixed action reuptake inhibitors (serotonin, norepinephrine, dopamine), 86t
moclobemide, 87t
monoamine oxidase inhibitors, 11, 85, 87t
motivational interviewing, 11b

nabilone/cannabis, 90t
narrative therapy, 11b
National Comprehensive Cancer Network (NCCN)
 anxiety management algorithm, 32f
 distress, defined, 4

distress guidelines, 5
distress management algorithm, 32f
distress management guidelines, 8, 10f
distress screening overview, 7b
Distress Thermometer and Problem List, 2, 4, 5, 7, 70, 109, 111
distress vulnerability periods, 6b
National Institute for Health and Care Excellence (NICE), 35
neuroleptics, 12b, 33
nonspecific distress, 7–8
norepinephrine-dopamine reuptake inhibitors (NRIs), 86t, 90t
nortriptyline, 87t

olanzapine, 18, 87t, 91t
  for adjustment disorders, 11
  for anxiety disorders, 18–19
  for depression, 94
  for insomnia in anxiety, depression, 85
  suicide risk and, 69
Omega 3, 90t
overgeneralization, 36t
oxazepam, 89t

panic disorder, 3, 16t, 19
paroxetine
  for anxiety, 86t
  for comorbid panic disorder, 19
  for depression, 86t
  discontinuation syndrome, 84b
  for generalized anxiety disorder, 19
  for PTSD, 19
Patient Health Questionnaire (PHQ-9), 27, 40, 111
patient's rights within the law, 71b
personalization, 36t
phenelzine, 87t
phobias
  in anxiety disorders, 3, 14

pharmacologic management, 98
specific phobia, 15, 16t, 92t
types of, 15
pindolol, 89t
posttraumatic stress disorder (PTSD), 3, 14, 15, 18, 19, 99
pregabalin, 89t, 98
problem-solving therapy, 35t, 37, 40
prochlorperazine, 18
professional issues, service implementation
  in anxiety disorder management, 20
  in demoralization, 59
  in depression, 39–40
  in suicide risk, 74
promethazine, 18
propanolol, 89t
psychiatric workup for distress, 6–7, 6b, 7b
psycho-educational interventions, 11b
psychopharmacologic options
  for adjustment disorders, 11–13, 99
  for anxiety disorders, 18–19, 86t–92t, 97–102
  for demoralization, 58
  for depression, 31, 33–35, 85, 86t–92t, 93–97
  for distress and anxiety, 18–19, 32f
  for suicide risk, 68–69, 69b, 70
psychostimulants, 31, 87t, 94–95
psychotherapeutic options
  for adjustment disorders, 9–11, 13
  for anxiety disorders, 18–20, 81, 104
  for demoralization, 44, 49, 50, 52, 53–57, 53–58
  for depression, 31, 32f, 35–39, 81, 104
  for suicide ideation, 69

questionnaires
  for adjustment disorders, 9

for anxiety, 18
for depression, 27, 28, 39–40, 111
for suicide risk, 67
quetiapine
  antidepressant effect of, 33
  for anxiety, 86t
  for depression, 86t, 94
  drug interactions, 103t
  for insomnia, 85
  side effects, 94
  for suicide risk, 69

reboxetine, 86t
reconstructing meaning and cognitive-analytic therapy, 11b
relaxation techniques
  for depression, 37
  description, 35t
  for distress management, 7
  effectiveness of, 37
  for insomnia, 19
  types of, 35t, 37, 102
risperidone, 18, 87t, 92t
RxList, drug interaction checker, 102

SAFE-T (Suicide Assessment Five-Step Evaluation and Triage), 112
SAM-e, 90t
schizophrenia, 62, 69, 74
seasonal affective disorder (SAD), 34
selective-norepinephrine reuptake inhibitors. See serotonin-norepinephrine reuptake inhibitors
selective serotonin reuptake inhibitors (SSRIs)
  for adjustment disorders, 11
  for anxiety, 86t
  for comorbid panic disorder, 19
  for depression, 33, 85, 86t
  discontinuation syndrome, 84, 85
  side effects, 33–34
  for suicide risk, 68, 69b

self-harm risk management, in suicidal patients, 71–74
serotonin-norepinephrine reuptake inhibitors (SNRIs)
- for adjustment disorders, 11
- for depression, 95
- efficacy, tolerability of, 93
- side effects, 33–34
- for suicide risk, 69b
- withdrawal recommendation, 34

serotonin syndrome, 12, 102
sertraline, 19, 86t, 93, 103t
SGAs. See antipsychotics, second-generation
"should" thinking, 36t
social anxiety disorder, 17t
specific
- phobia, 15, 16t, 92t
St. John's Wort, 90t
stress management, 18, 32f
substance abuse disorders, 62
substance/medication-induced anxiety disorder, 17t
Suicide Behaviors Questionnaire-Revised (SBQ-R), 112
Suicide Ideation and Risk Level Assessment, 112
suicide risk, 62–76
- assessment, 64–67, 67b, 71
- case study, 70
- demoralization and, 44
- diagnostic difficulties, 66
- differential diagnosis, 66
- efficacy/safety of psychotropic drugs, 69b
- inpatient management, 68b
- management of, 67–74, 75b
- patient capacity determination, 71–74
- of patients in the community, 74
- patient's rights within the law, 71b
- professional issues, service implementation, 74–76
- psychopharmacologic options, 68–69, 69b, 70
- psychotherapy options, 69
- rates data, 62
- risk factors, 62–63, 64b
- self-harm risk management, 71–74
- supportive-expressive therapy, 11b, 18, 35t, 55

sympathomimetics, 15
systematic desensitization, 19

T3/liothyronine, 88t
temazepam, 89t, 97
tranylcypromine, 87t
trazodone, 69, 85, 86t
triazolam, 19
tricyclic antidepressants (TCAs)
- for adjustment disorders, 11
- for anxiety, 87t
- cautions, 69b, 103t
- for depression, 87t, 93
- efficacy/safety in suicide ideation, 69b
- for insomnia, 93
- side effects, 34
triiodothyronine, 88t

U.S. Preventive Services Task Force, 27

valproate, 88t
venlafaxine
- for anxiety, 19, 86t
- for comorbid panic disorder, 19
- for depression, 68, 70, 86t, 97
- discontinuation syndrome, 84, 84b, 86t, 93
- drug interactions, 103b
- for generalized anxiety disorder, 19
- for hot flashes, 95b
- for suicide risk, 68, 70
vilazodone, 87t
vortioxetine, 87t, 94

worrying, chronic, 15

zaleplon, 19, 90t
zolpidem, 11, 19, 90t
zopiclone, 90t